W9-CEL-970

THE DECISION TREE

THE DECISION TREE

TAKING CONTROL OF YOUR HEALTH
IN THE NEW ERA OF PERSONALIZED MEDICINE

THOMAS GOETZ

Thomas Goetz

RODALE

This book is intended as a reference volume only, not as a medical manual. The information given here is designed to help you make informed decisions about your health. It is not intended as a substitute for any treatment that may have been prescribed by your doctor. If you suspect that you have a medical problem, we urge you to seek competent medical help.

Mention of specific companies, organizations, or authorities in this book does not imply endorsement by the author or publisher, nor does mention of specific companies, organizations, or authorities imply that they endorse this book, its author, or the publisher.

Internet addresses and telephone numbers given in this book were accurate at the time it went to press.

Portions of some chapters have appeared, in different form, in *Wired* and the *New York Times Magazine*.

© 2010 by Thomas Goetz

All rights reserved. No part of this publication may be reproduced or transmitted in any form or by any means, electronic or mechanical, including photocopying, recording, or any other information storage and retrieval system, without the written permission of the publisher.

Rodale books may be purchased for business or promotional use or for special sales. For information, please write to:
Special Markets Department, Rodale Inc., 733 Third Avenue, New York, NY 10017
Printed in the United States of America
Rodale Inc. makes every effort to use acid-free ⊗, recycled paper ☺.

Illustrations by Victor Krummenacher
Book design by Chris Rhoads

Library of Congress Cataloging-in-Publication Data

Goetz, Thomas.
The decision tree : taking control of your health in the new era of personalized medicine / Thomas Goetz.
        p.   cm.
Includes bibliographical references and index.
ISBN–13: 978–1–60529–729–3   hardcover
ISBN–10: 1–60529–729–1   hardcover
  1. Self-care, Health.   2. Medicine, Preventive.   3. Medical screening.
4. Medical technology.   I. Title.
    RA776.95.G64 2010
    613—dc22   2009038550

Distributed to the trade by Macmillan

2   4   6   8   10   9   7   5   3   1   hardcover

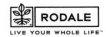

We inspire and enable people to improve their lives and the world around them

For more of our products visit rodalestore.com or call 800-848-4735

FOR WHITNEY,
REX, AND BUCK

Contents

Introduction

Every night, Laurie Fournier looks at a chart of the human body and makes a decision: where to stick the needle.

Like 400,000 other Americans, Laurie, a 48-year-old massage therapist living in a suburb of Minneapolis, has multiple sclerosis (MS), a disease classified as an autoimmune disorder, meaning one in which the body turns against itself. In the case of MS, the immune system targets the central nervous system, in particular the fatty sheath that covers each neuron. In someone with MS the immune system, which normally assaults damaged cells or invaders, perceives this sheath—known as myelin—as an antigen that must be destroyed. Alas, these myelin sheaths are not ordinary fat; they have the essential task of carrying electrical signals from nerve to nerve throughout the body. And so, as the immune system's T cells begin their attack, a person with MS may notice certain things starting to go wrong. His eyes might begin to twitch, he might have trouble pronouncing words, or he might simply feel off-balance. These symptoms can come and go in episodes, randomly enough that it typically takes years for someone to assemble the various symptoms into a pattern that leads to a diagnosis of MS.

There is no cure for MS, but there are treatments—drugs to slow down the immune system or distract the body from its self-destruction. In Laurie's case, a drug called Copaxone (glatiramer acetate) seems to act as a decoy to the T cells, drawing them away from the myelin and thus impeding the disease's progress. Like insulin for diabetics, Copaxone is delivered by regular self-administered injections. Learning the technique takes a certain amount of practice, particularly since Copaxone can cause some annoying side effects at the injection site, such as itching, swelling, lumps, and redness.

This is why Copaxone users like Laurie plan their shots using a chart that marks the body into a grid. This "shot journal" notes about 60 potential injection sites on the abdomen, arms, and legs. It's important, Laurie says, to follow a sequence and avoid putting today's shot too close to yesterday's or the day before's. "If you keep hitting the same spot, the tissue becomes fibrotic," she explains, making it difficult to flex the muscle. So before she goes to bed, she consults the chart, delivers the injection, and marks a box in the body grid with an X.

Laurie, who describes herself as an "information junkie," deals with these details with a blasé precision. MS can be an exhausting disease that weighs on people throughout the decades that they must live with it. But Laurie doesn't consider herself much different from anybody else. "Pretty much everybody I know over 45 has some kind of medical condition," she says. "Some people have had cataract surgery, or they have high cholesterol or diabetes. Everyone has something. And if everyone has something, that really levels the playing field."

Laurie is exactly right. When it comes to our health, we all have something we need to heed. Maybe it's a bum knee or a sore back, or perhaps it's something more serious, like cancer. It could be we've been diagnosed with a risk-based condition like high blood pressure that puts us in jeopardy of developing a more dangerous disease. Sure, some people are exceptions, those few who are in 100 percent perfect health today— in which case, well, something certainly looms for them in the future. The fact is that past a certain age, every one of us is made aware that his or her health is a variable, not a constant. At some point, health becomes complicated, something we must tend to, and often something scary.

And we learn that health demands that we make choices and compromises. But even before that happens, we need to be paying attention.

Laurie Fournier's circumstances—the gravity of her choices—might seem a world away from our own health concerns. Yes, we should exercise more, and we should eat better (and less). But by and large we may not think of health as an issue. We visit the doctor regularly and deal with the results when they come. We're doing fine. From this perspective, we'd define health as freedom from disease or illness. But that binary definition misses the subtle way we actually *experience* our health. It misses the multitude of other considerations, from our quality of life to our ability to meet a specific goal—be it to run a marathon or simply walk to the car—that go into caring for ourselves. And it misses the opportunity we all have to actually better our health, to improve the quality of our lives and pursue more ambitious goals. And in this regard, our health is very much like hers.

In truth, we are constantly making a series of decisions, some unconsciously, some with great intent, that combine to create our health. Some of these decisions can be easy: remembering to go to the dentist for an annual checkup, or opting to take a statin drug if we have high cholesterol. Others are exceedingly difficult and apt to provoke anxiety. Women with a high genetic risk of breast cancer, for instance, face a choice of whether to have a preemptive surgery or to begin drug treatment. Men diagnosed with prostate cancer typically choose between surgery or radiation treatment—both of which carry significant side effects—or decide to do nothing, hoping the cancer remains quiescent. Health is a constant negotiation between what we *want* to happen and what *may* happen. In health as in life, uncertainty is always part of the equation.

Medical science has made stupendous progress over the past 100 years. In 1910, polio and smallpox were common around the globe, crippling or killing millions of people. Today, vaccines have made the first almost unheard of and the second alive only in a few laboratories. In 1910, diabetes was a horrible disease that was treated with starvation, baths, and amputation; 30 percent of people with diabetes died from it.

Today, insulin injections and careful blood-sugar management have made it an entirely manageable disease. We are all infinitely better off for these innovations, and they are rightly hailed as miracles of science.

By and large, though, medical knowledge has been accessible only through an inefficient and cloistered health care system; our only entry point has been through the expertise of a physician. The education and training required to be a doctor is staggering, and physicians are rightly esteemed as an expert class of stature and influence. But the patient's role in his or her own care, ironically, has been an afterthought at best and a distraction at worst. Making medical decisions has been the physician's job, never our own. When we seek treatment, we often find ourselves lost, adrift in a poorly designed system that pushes us along quickly and officiously from the silo of one specialist to the next. We're told to always ask our doctors, but then we're consigned to less than 15 minutes of face time in an office visit. When we seek out information, we get lost in a muddle of contradictory studies and imprecise advice. Too often, we come to realize that the best opportunity for action is already gone, having come before we even thought about our health. All in all, this is not the way to stay healthy. And it's not the way a 21st-century society, with a health care system steeped in science, should treat its citizens.

THIS BOOK IS ABOUT HOW we can make better choices for our health. Today, we have the opportunity to engage with our health more prudently, more strategically, and more effectively. We can engage through new science and technologies, tapping the best practices of genetics, behavioral science, information technology, and even each other. We can make sense of the babel of data to craft a personal strategy for making the best choices that lead to the best outcomes. We can take a central role in our health and be the better for it.

The central organizing principle of this approach is a *Decision Tree*, a system that maps out our options, factors in all the relevant information and our backgrounds and statuses, and guides us toward the best possible decision, whether the choice is to take a screening test or not, how to best respond to a diagnosis, or whether to try a new drug. A Decision Tree is a simple idea—many of us, after all, learned to draw them in the form of flowcharts in fourth or fifth grade. But in an age of too much information and too little guidance, they're a handy way to think about our options and take some control over our health. On a basic level, a Decision Tree is simply a tool that nudges us to think through our options, to act consciously and with consideration. And it puts us in the central role as decision makers—not the doctor, the insurance company, or a hospital administrator. By factoring in our family histories, our good and bad habits, and, ultimately, the conditions we need to ward off or treat, using a Decision Tree approach can maximize our efforts to push ill health, and ultimately death, as far into the future as possible. It's a powerful way to think about our health.

Decision Trees are already all around us. They're common in engineering and industry, where they're known as algorithms. The pharmaceutical industry uses them to predict drug safety in clinical trials. Computer scientists use them to root out patterns of credit card fraud. They're even used by civil engineers to plan streetlight patterns and map out school bus routes. And over the past decade or so, they've become a common tool in medicine, used by doctors to weigh the effects of different interventions and factor in various probabilities for various treatments. In these cases, Decision Trees can be complicated structures laden with mathematics and computer science. But they needn't be only for the experts. A Decision Tree can be as straightforward as writing down the pros and cons and noting the risks and benefits *before* we act.

Think of it this way: Health is, in many respects, a system of inputs and outputs. The inputs start with the huge number of choices we make every day that have a great influence on our health: what we choose to eat, whether or not we exercise, how much we sleep, whether we heed our doctors' orders. These choices combine with other inputs, things that we may not even consider to be medical information and that we probably know much more about than our doctors—like our family history, where we live, our jobs, our stress levels, and so on. All of these inputs together create one primary output that is unique to us alone: our health, for good or for ill. This is our Decision Tree. This is the opportunity before us. The more we're conscious of these inputs, the more often we take the time to think them through and maybe even write them down, the better are our chances of making the best decisions and having the best lives. The ideas and science and stories inside this book are meant to help each of us grasp that opportunity.

So what does a Decision Tree look like? Throughout this book, I'll present different people's Decision Trees as a way to make explicit the choices they face and how they're weighing their situations. Sometimes actually putting pen to paper and sketching out a Decision Tree can be helpful. But chiefly, a Decision Tree is a concept, a frame of mind that helps us think about our health, a process that should begin years before it typically does.

THERE ARE THREE FUNDAMENTAL PRINCIPLES of making smart health choices. They are common rules that can make a decision about whether to have a screening test or undergo surgery or begin a new diet more likely to result in a good outcome.

THE FIRST RULE: EARLY IS BETTER THAN LATE

It's well known that the earlier medicine begins to treat disease, the better the outcome. And when we treat disease before it happens—by going after risks rather than symptoms—we can do even better. These days, "acting early" means that by learning our genetic predispositions—starting, when possible, at birth (or even before)—we can modify our choices in life. "Acting early" means that when we're at a higher-than-average risk for something like colon cancer, we'll go ahead and have a colonoscopy regularly (screening, after all, is better than surgery). And if something is found, treatment will be a much simpler and less invasive process, with far better odds of success.

Acting early sounds like the obvious path to take, but it's far from the norm in health care today. Indeed, more than 70 percent of the

A Decision Tree for Health

Thinking actively about our health concerns and choices not only improves our decision making—it can improve our well-being. Here's a sample of how a Decision Tree can start with some basic family history.

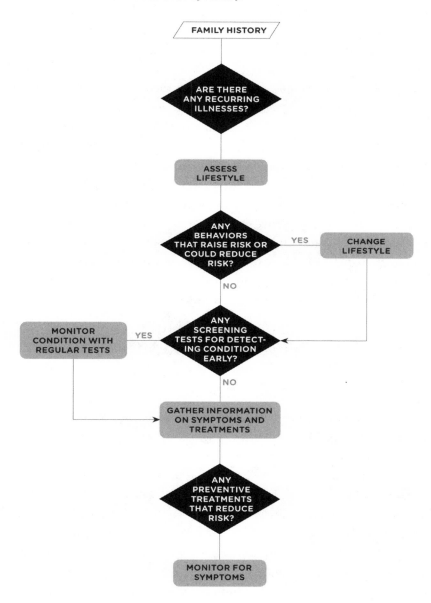

$2 trillion spent on health care in the United States goes to chronic disease treatments and late-stage interventions. This is the status quo of health care today, and, like any status quo, it won't be easy to change. Most doctors, as I'll explain, are compensated for exactly the wrong things: diagnosing and treating disease, rather than preventing and warding off illness. Often, if there's nothing wrong, there's nothing a physician can bill for. Some screening procedures are covered by insurance, but not enough—and don't even think about trying to get a genetic test covered without an exceptional reason.

Acting early is hard for individuals as well. We Americans have proven ourselves to be awfully slow about engaging with our health before something goes wrong. Screening rates for simple procedures that are known to improve outcomes—regular testing for colon cancer for example—are consistently low. And the rising obesity rate—two-thirds of Americans are now overweight, with 30 percent of that number qualifying as obese—shows that we're not good at taking preemptive action on health matters. Obesity can open the door to many worse conditions, such as type 2 diabetes, heart disease, and stroke. Acting early, in other words, can be more difficult than it sounds.

THE SECOND RULE:
LET DATA DO THE WORK

Data can be a scary word. It brings to mind statistics, formulas, and lots and lots of numbers, the stuff we thought we left behind back in calculus class. But data is very much the foundation of medical science, where fealty to scientific rigor has made possible so many of the treatments and cures we count on today. In the past decade or so, this faith in data has spread to the doctor's office with the rise of evidence-based medicine, which insists that a caregiver's every decision be based on clinically valid research. And, as we'll see, now there are even opportunities for individuals to heed more complicated data as well, to be guided by statistics and true probabilities to make better-informed, smarter decisions.

There's another sense in which data can play a part in our health decisions: the data that we generate ourselves. More than just the workup from a hospital or doctor's office, we generate a constant stream of information. It's in our diets, our exercising, our moods, our DNA. And just as the recommendation engines at Amazon.com and Netflix.com use our customer histories to help us choose the right book or movie (or, at eHarmony, the right spouse), this data constitutes powerful information that can help inform our health decisions. This data can create a feedback loop for better health. Knowing our personal data gives us a baseline from which to evaluate our future health, revealing whether we're improving or slacking off. It can also be used to fine-tune the risks for disease, augmenting the population-level numbers we're all given (the 36 percent risk of developing heart disease in America, or the 8 percent risk of developing type 2 diabetes) to create personalized risk models that tell us what each of us should prioritize.

This drive toward data, of course, means that each of us must become more comfortable with predictions and probabilities, more at ease with weighing our options based on statistical risk rather than symptoms. Navigating our way through the data can challenge the best of us. But as I'll explain in Chapter 1, research shows that, when numbers are properly framed, ordinary people are more capable of handling them than many medical professionals assume. What's more, research has shown that in many of the medical decisions we're faced with—how to interpret a test, how to decide upon a treatment, or when to move to a different treatment—trusting data can improve our decision making and our outcomes.

THE THIRD RULE: TRUST IN OPENNESS

In the technology world, *openness* and *transparency* have become the new buzzwords as the principles of collaboration and sharing have spread from open-source software to Wikipedia to Yelp.com. Bringing openness to health care, on the other hand, sounds like a less obvious proposition. Sharing our personal information with strangers sounds downright risky. After all, doesn't more openness mean less privacy?

The answer is both no (not necessarily) and yes (but it's nothing to worry about). The truth is that our personal information, including our health information, is a currency, something we can exchange with others to create new, more powerful information. Facebook and Twitter have changed the notion of privacy and fostered a much more open display of personal information that has yielded all sorts of benefits in terms of friendship, entertainment, and even political change. The same sort of structure, sharing, and cooperation can benefit health care as well.

At the very least, bringing more openness to our decision making means demanding more transparency from our physicians. We shouldn't have to ask for copies of our medical records or test results, and when we do, they should be provided without hesitation. Our doctors should be urged and, indeed, expected to fully integrate patients into making decisions on medical care. Openness, not paternalism or isolation, should be the default mode in health care.

Openness can offer even more in the form of collaborative research. Individuals are now able to share information about their genomes to create new bodies of information about genetic risk, and they're contributing information about their drug dosages and symptoms to build information banks that can help everyone maintain their health or treat disease. This is how Laurie Fournier became such an expert about Copaxone injections—by sharing her information and experiences and learning from others at a Web site called PatientsLikeMe (I discuss the company at length in Chapter 10). Yes, this means contributing private information, but only with full knowledge of what we're giving up and what it's being used for. Anonymity is always an option. But openness can have another powerful benefit for individuals facing health decisions. Openness reduces isolation. It helps to know that someone else has faced the same quandary we have. That can be a powerful medicine all its own.

THESE THREE PRINCIPLES aren't just smart ideas or vogue philosophies. They have all been scientifically associated with better health. Early detection of ovarian cancer, for instance, can boost the odds of survival to upwards of 90 percent, a huge leap from the mere 15 percent survival rate for a cancer found in the last stages (I get into this in Chapter 7). Tracking and monitoring our own data has been strongly associated with good health, not only because it makes it easier to lose weight or lower our cholesterol levels, but also because it seems to offer us a sense of control that contributes to better health and well-being (I'll explain more about this notion of control in Chapter 1). And openness has become a resonant topic in medical research: Having strong social networks has been linked to success in quitting smoking, losing weight, and modifying other behaviors (as I'll discuss in Chapter 4).

What's more, there's also ample evidence that using a Decision Tree approach can, in general, have a positive impact on health. Research has demonstrated that individuals who are actively involved in making their own medical decisions have significantly better outcomes than those who rely only on their doctors to make the calls. In other words, simply by participating in the process, we're more likely to have better results. The more we mind our health, the more we take charge of it (rather than being subject to it), the better our outcomes. This is the power of the Decision Tree.

THE IDEA FOR THIS BOOK came to me a few years ago, during a hectic period when I was simultaneously working as an editor at *Wired* magazine in San Francisco and studying for a master's degree in public health at the University of California, Berkeley. Early every morning, I would drive across the Bay Bridge to the campus, where I'd wrestle with epidemiology, biostatistics, and health economics. I was captivated by the discipline of public health, its deference to data, and its mandate to think in the largest possible scale—populations, not individuals. Public health, I learned, had been preaching the mantra of prevention long before it became fashionable. After all, the cheapest, most efficient way to improve the public health is to keep the public healthy in the first place.

This approach was best described to me by S. Leonard Syme, PhD, a legendary figure at Berkeley who pioneered the study of social causes of disease. In a lecture one morning, Dr. Syme challenged his students with a scenario: People are traveling in their cars along a highway, only to find that the road heads directly off a cliff. Not surprisingly, this creates a pileup at the cliff's bottom, with all sorts of injuries and fatalities. "So where do you put the hospital?" Dr. Syme asked the class. It was, of course, a trick question. Conventional medicine tends to build its hospitals at the base of the cliff, where the bodies are. But the answer from a public health perspective would be to avoid building a hospital at all. Better to move the highway, or build a bridge, or somehow intervene *before* people plunge into the abyss. Sure, it sounds obvious, but then again, if it's obvious, why does preventive medicine get such short shrift? It's a simple lesson, but a profound one.

After attending my classes each morning, I'd race back across the bridge to San Francisco and shift my attention to my job at *Wired*, where we chronicle the profound impact technology is having throughout business and culture. At the time, Silicon Valley was in the early throes of what's called Web 2.0—a new generation of Internet tools that draw on an individual's own participation and collaboration to create a highly personalized online experience. Facebook, MySpace, and Twitter are all spawn of the Web 2.0 boom. The power of personalization was taking off.

As months of this back-and-forth went by, I was struck by the unfortunate disconnect between the public health world and the technology world. After all, technology and public health both share an appetite for scale—the idea that an innovation becomes more powerful as its cost drops and accessibility increases. In technology, this is known as Moore's law, and it's what makes digital cameras and high-definition TVs and so many other digital gadgets cost half as much this year as they did last year. Public health is all about scale, too—vaccines are the perfect cheap technology, as are simple, cheap screening tests like mammography and blood tests. But many corners of the public health world harbor a suspicion of technology, a worry that bells and whistles distract from the goal of bringing health to the maximum number of people. In part, there's good reason for doubt. Modern medicine has too often gotten technology wrong, letting it drive costs up rather than down. A major factor in the $2 trillion–and–climbing the United States spends on health care annually is the appetite for newer, *more expensive* devices and instruments. These technologies don't scale, and so they're often out of reach for too many people.

But there's an opportunity, I began to realize, to combine the lessons of technology and the rigor of public health. These same Internet tools could be adapted to filter and tailor the great insights of medical research to individuals' situations, helping them make the best decisions at the right time—*before* they plunge off the cliff into poor health. What's more, these technologies offer scale, so they can be used by a great number of people for little increase in cost. The impact wouldn't just be a healthier person here or there; the potential is to help *lots* of people.

It turned out that some folks are way ahead of me. Here and there, entrepreneurs have been creating tools that could organize and gather information to benefit individuals' health. Some people are looking at genetic science, figuring out ways to give people a look at how their DNA makeup can help predict future health issues. Others are creating data-gathering tools that let people easily keep track of everything they eat in order to more effectively lose weight. And still others are building Web sites for people with chronic diseases, places where they can organize their drug regimens and symptomatology to keep abreast of the best treatments. In this book, I visit many of these innovators, from giants like Microsoft and Kaiser Permanente to startups like Tethys Bioscience and CureTogether.com. The seeds of a Decision Tree approach are already out there and spreading quickly.

IN NOVEMBER 2008, *Operations Research,* an eminent academic journal in the somewhat obscure world of applied mathematics and statistical analysis, published a paper with the provocative title "Personal Decisions Are the Leading Cause of Death."

The paper was the work of Ralph Keeney, a professor at Duke University's business school. Drawing on a rather ordinary pool of data gathered from, among other places, the Centers for Disease Control and Prevention (CDC), Keeney's conclusion was nonetheless shocking.

Among people between 15 and 64 years old, fully 55 percent of all deaths in the United States are attributable to personal decisions. That, Keeney argued, is an increase from just 5 percent of deaths a century ago. At first glance, it looked as if Keeney had spotted an epidemic of stupidity. But, in fact, what Keeney had classified as personal decisions spanned the breadth of human behavior: Yes, accidents, but also smoking, poor diet, too much alcohol, and so on. These are the bad decisions that, in Keeney's estimation, are leading so many of us—indeed, *most* of us—to our doom.

The paper caused a bit of a stir, and *Newsweek*'s headline was typical of the reaction: "America's Top Killer: Us." But what's notable about Keeney's research isn't really his conclusions; after all, all the CDC data are widely available, and nearly all of these trends have been apparent for decades. Certainly it came as little news to the public health community that bad behavior can cost lives. What *is* novel is the way Keeney approaches the data, the way he talks about it. As a risk analyst, rather than an epidemiologist or an MD, Keeney simply frames the data in his terms: He sees these as economic calculations as much as medical ones. From his point of view, our health is the result of the mental cost-benefit decisions we all make—choices that ultimately lead to our deaths more often than not. "These are decisions worthy of thought," he says. "We should get people to think a little more clearly about their alternatives." And *that* is new—the idea that health is a decision-making problem as much as a health care problem. That new prism puts these familiar statistics in an entirely new and penetrating light. For the majority of the things that actually turn out to kill us, Keeney is telling us, we actually have a *choice* in the matter.

Keeney's paper reflects the awesome power of our decisions in our health. We are the greatest arbiters, more than our doctors or surgeons or even the insurance companies, of how we will live and how healthy we will be. These are the roots, if you will, of a Decision Tree approach: acknowledging and then exploiting the role that our own choices play in our health. Throughout this book, I've tried to follow Keeney's lead and flush out where we have decisions to make, even when we wouldn't ordinarily think of it. By thinking about our health as a series of choices, some mundane and others grave, it's my hope to point the way toward *better* choices.

Accordingly, I have organized the book into three parts, following the three phases of health as most people experience it. Part I, Prediction and Prevention, involves our first opportunities to engage with and influence our health—before we get a disease. This book will argue that DNA can be a library for self-knowledge, but I won't pretend that the science doesn't have a long way to go before it starts to guide the courses of our lives. I'll consider the paradox of behavior change—how we don't do what we know we should—a riddle that has stumped physicians and philosophers going back to Aristotle. And I'll check in on Weight Watchers—yes, Weight Watchers—which has honed an approach to behavior modification that elegantly demonstrates how quantitative information and social networks can be instrumental in improving health. As Keeney's paper makes clear, our first decisions can be the most important ones, and at this early point we want to anticipate disease and pursue our lives starting from the best possible circumstances.

Part II, Diagnosis and Detection, starts where most of us actually begin to take our health seriously—after we've been diagnosed with something. In contemporary medicine, diagnosis has come to mean two things. On the one hand, it retains its original sense of finding a biological disease early in its course, which I discuss in terms of screening tests and the early detection of cancer. But diagnosis increasingly concerns something else as well, a state that exists in a definitional sense more than a biological one. This is the realm of predisease, the idea of fixing a diagnosis now in order to avoid a worse one later.

Part III tackles Care and Treatment—that point where most of us will, inevitably, arrive. I'll explain why most pharmaceuticals are surprisingly ineffective, making smart decisions about drug treatments difficult, and I'll review new efforts to better target drugs to individuals. But treatment is about more than drugs. It's mostly about making a multitude of smaller decisions, each of which takes on higher stakes once disease is diagnosed. And I'll explore how the power of openness is bringing patients together to create powerful new data sets that can improve treatments—and even yield new science.

Along the way, this book will touch on everything from genetics to neuroscience. We'll visit anatomy labs in Renaissance Italy and head west across the 19th-century American frontier. And we'll meet real people who are facing tough decisions, and talk with others, like Laurie Fournier, who have already braved the waters. Their Decision Trees can serve as models for our own.

What I *won't* dwell on is miracle drugs that have shown incredible results in lab mice or some high-tech "future of medicine" that's unlikely ever to happen. Real personalized medicine should begin long before we're faced with pharmacology; the opportunity for us to customize our health care as individuals should begin long before we ever get sick. Anybody who has had reason to spend any time in a hospital recently knows as well as I do that the future of medicine is a long, long way off. Medicine is a messy, disorganized, reactionary affair, and I won't pretend otherwise.

But reality still has plenty going for it, starting with tools and technologies that can help sort this mess into something more useful and effective for ordinary people. A Decision Tree approach doesn't assume that we're about to enter a golden age of perfect medicine. Nor do I assume that putting individuals at the center of their health care means they're on their own. This isn't do-it-yourself medicine. Doctors remain an integral and essential part of effective health care. But they are no longer the only actors on the stage.

This is no quick fix. What I'm writing about demands that we adjust to more complexity, that we take on more responsibility in ambiguous circumstances. In the short term, at least, it could be a more confusing process. But my hope is that readers will come away armed with ideas and strategies for dealing with what are often the most confusing and scary moments in our lives. My mission is to offer a structure—the Decision Tree—that diminishes uncertainty and allows us to make better choices for ourselves at the right time. A Decision Tree can bear the fruit of a better life.

PART I

Prediction and Prevention

1

Living by Numbers

How a Lot of Science and a Little Self-Awareness Can Give You Control of Your Health

I.

AVIATION HAS KITTY HAWK. Biology has the Galápagos Islands. And medicine, or more specifically preventive medicine, has Framingham, Massachusetts.

A small city of 65,000 people about 20 miles due west of Boston, Framingham appears at first an indistinct patch of New England suburbia. Take Exit 13 off the Massachusetts Turnpike, and you'll drive past the usual temples of American sprawl: a Shopper's World shopping center (among the first malls built in the United States), a Super Stop & Shop grocery store, and a Lowe's, all built in the same squat, stuccoed style and painted in the same tan-to-taupe palette that characterizes the rest of American consumerland. As you drive along Highway 9 toward Framingham's center, it's easy to miss the original town. Even the arrow on the sign that points toward "Downtown Framingham" makes only a half-hearted gesture in the right direction, as if it can't decide whether or not to recommend the place. But make the turn, and the town starts to hint at its more dignified origins; pass the requisite Revolutionary War statue, and you'll reach the stately brick and stone buildings of what must have once been a thriving town center. These days, though, like many neglected downtowns outdone by the interstate, Framingham's center is dotted with empty storefronts and tinged with sad neglect.

None of this hints at why Framingham actually matters. In the years after World War II, when the town was a far smaller place with a population of just around 28,000, Framingham became the epicenter of what would become one of the great experiments in medicine—an experiment that is still running quietly today. In 1948, the National Heart Institute chose Framingham as the place that would reveal the causes of heart disease.

At the time, the idea of studying a disease by studying a population was an altogether novel concept, and an urgent one. In the first decades of the 20th century, most infectious diseases were eliminated from the United States and other industrialized nations. Cholera, diphtheria, typhoid, malaria, tuberculosis—all the diseases that had plagued mankind for centuries were largely banished from our shores as vaccines, antibiotics, and sanitation did their work. The result was profound: The average life span for an American male increased from 46 years in 1900 to 61 by 1940, while the average for women increased from 48 to 65.

But as remarkable as the elimination of infectious disease was, it didn't eliminate disease entirely. In fact, it revealed a new, unknown sort of disease, one that seemed to fester beneath the surface until it struck. A stunning 36 percent of Americans died of just two conditions in 1940: heart disease and stroke. But unlike with tuberculosis, it wasn't possible to lay the blame on a single pathogen. Medicine in postwar America had almost no idea what caused heart attacks or strokes or the other fatal events related to heart disease. They just happened. It was as if by eliminating epidemics of infectious diseases, medicine had unwittingly allowed new epidemics to kill thousands of other people.

By singling out Framingham, the National Heart Institute (known today as the National Heart, Lung, and Blood Institute) was taking a bold step: It would investigate heart disease as thoroughly, ambitiously, and successfully as the nation had fought World War II. Framingham then was just as much an Everytown, USA, as it is today. It had a mix of ethnic backgrounds: Irish, Greek, Polish, Italian. Its inhabitants smoked, worked in factories (GM opened a new plant in town in 1948), and, like other Americans, considered meat and potatoes a balanced diet. And when television came to town in 1948, they began to watch TV as well. They were, in other words, entirely typical citizens of postwar America.

The Framingham Heart Study, as it's called, began by recruiting as many townspeople as possible until it had enrolled 5,209 citizens—half of all of Framingham's adults, and nearly 20 percent of the total population. These citizens filled out a long questionnaire about their lifestyle, habits, and health; they tried to remember what their parents and grandparents had died of. They stripped down to their underwear and were given a thorough physical, including measuring their blood pressure and their lung capacity. A blood sample was taken and sent to the lab for tests. And every 2 years, these 5,209 citizens were called back for more poking, prodding, and reevaluation. The study has continued ever since. In 1971, it expanded to begin tracking a second generation of Framingham citizens—5,124 sons and daughters and their spouses of the original subjects. And in 2002, a third generation was signed up, 4,095 grandchildren. In Framingham, being one of the cohort is a point of family pride.

The size, ambition, and duration of the Framingham study—calling on thousands of townspeople and tracking them and their children and their children's children for more than 60 years—makes Framingham not an Everytown at all, but an exceptional experiment in science. The resulting pool of data has yielded insights into the human condition that were, prior to the study, entirely mysterious. The Framingham data have led to more than 1,200 published research papers, science that has broken ground on cholesterol and smoking and heart failure. It's because of Framingham that we know cigarettes increase the risk of heart disease. It's because of Framingham that we know high blood pressure can lead to stroke. And if not for Framingham, we'd have no idea that some cholesterol is good for you and some is bad. And it's not just heart disease. The Framingham data have been used to study osteoporosis, breast cancer, Alzheimer's disease, arthritis—even sleep and happiness.

Most of all, Framingham, more than any other piece of research, has created the concept of health risks, the idea that behind every chronic disease lies a certain chance of developing that disease. It has given us the idea that we can and should anticipate disease, and that we might be able to identify what leads to chronic disease just as we try to identify the bacteria or pathogens that lead to infectious diseases. Indeed, the very term *risk factors* comes out of Framingham. Blood pressure, body mass index, cholesterol, triglyceride level—all these metrics today reflect the essential research gathered in the Framingham study.

This concept of risk is integral to the way our society tries to improve health. On a population level, reducing risk is the cornerstone of public health, and in your doctor's office, identifying individual risk factors is the backbone of preventive care. The study has changed not only our understanding of heart disease but also our understanding of how science should be practiced. The Framingham approach—population research—is now standard practice in public health, the basic framework of the science of epidemiology.

The Framingham Heart Study itself is run out of a building about a mile from downtown, a squat, two-level complex painted in the same shade of taupe as the malls near the freeway. Aside from that building, the only public acknowledgments of the town's significance are street signs posted here and there that hail Framingham as the Town That Changed America's Heart. But it's no exaggeration to add that it's the town that changed our concept of health as well.

IT'S A PLEASANT SPRING EVENING in San Francisco, and a group of supremely self-obsessed people has gathered in a downtown office to compare notes—very, very specific and thorough notes. This group tracks pretty much anything and everything that one can imagine measuring, counting, or calculating about the human body. Blood pressure, weight, exercise, sleep, mood, menstruation—these folks track it all, down to the gram, the second, the microliter. Welcome to the Quantified Self monthly meet up, a group of people who believe that, in the future, our data will say more about us than anything. And they want to get to that future first.

The meeting begins with some chatting over beer and chips, and then the crowd of about 40 people grab seats and listen to a series of brief presentations. One by one, people stand up and chronicle their chronicling. One man recounts his struggle with sleep apnea and how tracking his sleep patterns has become, for him, a matter of great urgency. "I was having about 48 episodes a night," he tells the group. "That's classified as severe. That amount could be fatal." After surgery, he says, he's down to about 40 episodes—better, but still in the danger zone.

Next, a married couple steps forward to share how they've been tracking their relationship. "We can count the frequency of having sex," the woman says. "But we haven't been able to find another quantitative metric to assess our relationship." She notes that the frequency of intercourse goes up when her weight goes down, and vice versa.

Another woman, by her count, is tracking 40 metrics on a daily basis: her sleep, her weight, her caloric intake, her exercise quantity and duration, her supplements, her headaches and nausea, the length of time she works, the time she spends with her kids, and six separate factors that correspond to mood. In the data, she says, she finds order and some calm. "When I don't get anything out of it anymore, when it starts to be a net negative, then I'll stop. But for now I find it helpful, and I'm learning about myself," she says. "I've learned that weight is an issue for me, and that I should exercise more. And I've learned that I'm a pretty good mother. These are worthwhile insights."

To be fair, this crowd isn't really obsessed (at least not all of them). More accurately, they are passionate believers that there is real meaning, quantifiable meaning, to be found in everyday life. They believe that in our daily actions of living and breathing we are shedding data all the time, whether we're aware of it or not, and that by capturing this data stream and analyzing it, we might grasp some insight. In approaching life by the numbers, they have found some new way to engage with their lives.

It is, to say the least, an interesting group of people. Yes, this being San Francisco, many of them could be described as nerdy. There are beards and stickered laptops and discussions about experiment design and open-source software. This is perhaps to be expected. The Quantified Self folks are, in the jargon of technology, classic early adopters: people who throw themselves into an experiment with numbers and gadgets, a group that enjoys playing around with possibility and tinkering with what might be done. They are geeking out, in other words, just like the guys who stand in line for iPhones and then rush home and take them apart to see how they're made. Except in this case, the iPhones are their own bodies.

The iPhone, in fact, plays a significant part in the Quantified Self experiment. There are dozens of applications, or apps—little software programs—that can be loaded onto an iPhone to help you track your weight or your exercise or your glucose level or your nutritional intake. And there are dozens of other gadgets and Web sites that likewise offer to help track this number or quantify that variable. There is Fuelly, a Web site that lets any driver turn into a "hypermiler," wringing every possible mile from a tank of gas. There is Tweet What You Eat, a service that lets people Twitter about what they've consumed (the tweets are entered into a personal database). There's Wakoopa, which tracks certain Web sites you visit. And Garmin, the global positioning system (GPS) tools company, has MotionBased, a GPS-enabled mapping system and exercise calculator for bicyclists. The Quantified Self crowd uses all of these tools and more with an enthusiasm most of us save for our hobbies or our relationships.

The Quantified Self folks sense an opportunity at hand: the wide availability of tools and cheap technology to measure and save most anything you can think of. Not all of the data will have meaning, but the point, at this early stage, isn't necessarily to start drawing conclusions, it's simply to gather the information. They're turning everything into a possible input. And what are the outputs? They'll turn up in due time.

AROUND THE CORNER from Number 10 Downing Street, the British prime minister's residence, is Whitehall Street, the epicenter of the UK government. Whitehall is lined with offices; the Treasury building is just down from the Foreign Office, the Department of Health is across the street, and so on down the road. Every day, Whitehall Street is packed with workers—bureaucrats and diplomats, secretaries and sanitation workers—going about the business of government. Indeed, in the United Kingdom, "Whitehall" is as synonymous with "government" as "Washington" is in the United States. And that explains the name given to the Whitehall studies, two landmark pieces of public health research that provide an unusual perspective on the variety of factors that result in our health.

In 1967, just as the Framingham study was turning up its early conclusions about heart disease, a team of researchers from the London School of Hygiene and Tropical Medicine and University College London arrived on Whitehall Street to take a different crack at the same problem. The scientists, led by Michael Marmot, PhD, and Geoffrey Rose, wanted to know not *what* caused heart disease, but *who* was most at risk for it. They recruited more than 18,000 men from the British civil service (the agency that employs all the workers of Whitehall Street) between the ages of 40 and 64, when most heart attacks seemed to happen. These were the bookkeepers and administrators, the janitors and messengers that kept the government humming along, as well as the higher-level ministers and officials.

At the time, Britain was still a highly stratified society, marked by finely measured and codified class distinctions. The civil service was an especially perfect microcosm of this structure; as Dr. Marmot described it, it was "exquisitely stratified," like a bank or an insurance company or any "big white-collar corporation, only more so." This stratification made Whitehall an ideal place to examine what role status might play in health—especially since everyone had equal access to health care, provided via the National Health Service.

The 18,000 men were first given a medical examination, with particular attention being paid to their histories and known risks for cardiovascular disease. Then they were segmented into five groups based on their professional status. There was an executive grade at the top, then a professional grade, an administrative, a clerical, and finally an "other" category, which consisted of those of the lowest status (mostly unskilled laborers). For the next 7 years, these men were tracked. They were weighed, quizzed about their smoking, given periodic electrocardio-grams to measure their heart function, and so forth. But in the very first year, a trend quickly emerged: Those in the lowest social categories—the clerical workers and the "other" workers—were dying of heart disease in much greater numbers, while those in the highest social categories—the executive, professional, and administrative grades—were signifi-cantly more likely to remain alive. As the years went on, this trend became even more pronounced, so much so that those at the bottom end of the ladder were *four times* more likely to die of heart disease than those at the top, the study found. Clearly, there was something unhealthy about being at the bottom.

But what was it? All the men were about the same age, so age couldn't be a factor. There were, however, several other factors that did closely track the divergence. One of these was height; the administrative class was much taller, and heart disease seemed to afflict those shorter than 5 feet 6 inches much more than it did those over 6 feet. Similarly, those in the highest-risk groups tended to weigh more than those in the low-risk groups. Their habits differed as well. Men in the lower grades smoked more and ate poorer diets than those in the upper grades. And the health metrics already associated with heart disease—high blood pressure and elevated blood glucose level—were likewise worse in the lower grades.

In other words, all of the known risk factors for heart disease (the ones coming out of Framingham) were greater among those with lower social status. That was an interesting but not entirely surprising conclu-sion. It made sense that those with poorer health habits died of heart disease more often, and it made sense that those at the bottom of the social pyramid had more of those bad habits. That's the way of the world, in Britain as in the United States as in nearly everywhere else.

But that wasn't the end of it. When the researchers adjusted their numbers and factored out the discrepancies caused by known risk fac-tors, they still saw a huge gap. Smoking and diet and blood pressure and so on accounted for many of the deaths by heart disease, but far from all of them. Indeed, after crunching the numbers (what statisticians call con-trolling for those risk factors), the researchers could account for only

40 percent of the deaths by heart disease. For the other 60 percent of cases, something *unexplained* was killing people, and disproportionately killing those on the bottom rungs of society. Indeed, a man's social class was the *strongest* risk factor for heart disease, higher than even whether or not he smoked or was overweight. And a man in the lowest status group still had more than twice the risk of dying of heart disease. There was a clear and pronounced connection between class and disease. But there was no clear explanation for that connection.

In the first papers announcing their results, published in the late 1970s, Dr. Marmot and Rose put on the table a range of alternative explanations for the discrepancy. It could be genetic factors or unmeasured nutritional differences. They even suggested that inbreeding among the upper classes might have a protective effect. But in the ensuing years, Dr. Marmot began to pursue an alternative explanation: that the social status of the worker was in and of itself the determining factor, because it intensified the stresses of the workplace. Those with a lower status lacked control over their work. Their job was to do other people's bidding, not their own. They could not control their destiny. In his book *The Status Syndrome*, Dr. Marmot offers an example: "How many times have you called the telephone company, the airline, the bank, the insurance company, and, in exasperation, asked to speak to the frontline person's supervisor? You do this because the discretion of the lower-status person to make decisions is limited." The higher their status, the more control people had. And this small amount of authority—this thwarted need to control our own destinies—struck Dr. Marmot as perhaps the largest of all the risk factors for ill health.

"Control over destiny" doesn't exactly have the ring of a highly scientific term. It's not the sort of thing that can be readily measured or quantified (though in subsequent research, Dr. Marmot did develop ways for people to self-report their sense of control at the workplace). But it makes a certain visceral sense. We all know what it feels like to be in control, to be at the top of the pyramid. And we all know the opposite feeling, of being at the mercy of other people's decisions and whims. One is a feeling of confidence, of command, of vitality—it's the sort of thing we mean when we talk about "flow" and "instinct"—while the other is a feeling of helplessness and inconsequence and, at its worst, despair. In one we guide our own courses, we are the stewards of our decisions, the masters of our own fates. In the other, we are at fate's whim.

II.

WHAT ARE WE TO DRAW from the above? What do Framingham, Whitehall, and the Quantified Self crowd tell us about health? Consider their lessons collectively. Take the idea of health risks from Framingham, combine it with the powerful tools for self-tracking utilized by Quantified Self, and perhaps we can create the sense of control that Whitehall identified. In other words, by paying heed to our health and taking advantage of tools for self-monitoring, feedback, and community, perhaps we can empower our own actions and skirt the disease risks that life throws at us. Perhaps our health isn't fated, after all.

On its face, this may seem like an obvious notion. Surely this must already be the modus operandi of medicine. But it's not. In fact, health and medicine are practiced in pretty much the *opposite* way today. Just think of the way you receive most health information: It's a stern list of dos and don'ts—don't smoke, do get more exercise, and for God's sake do eat your vegetables. We have the surgeon general's warnings on cigarettes and health warnings for pregnant women in parking garages. We ban trans fats and stigmatize butterfat. Drug companies barrage us with direct-to-consumer advertising that, on one page, promises to end all our problems and, in tiny print on the next page, discloses all the dire side effects that may come along for the ride. Health information comes at us in a flood of warnings, research, and findings that make life seem like a walk through a minefield. Eventually we're going to miss a warning sign and take one wrong step.

That's pretty much the conversation on health risks today. The medical establishment has largely missed the lesson of the Whitehall studies and much subsequent research: that control matters. We are told what to do, but we are not given the tools to measure or assess our own progress. We have little control over our own destinies.

The Declining Number of Primary Care Doctors

Each year, more medical school graduates choose to become specialists instead of primary care physicians.

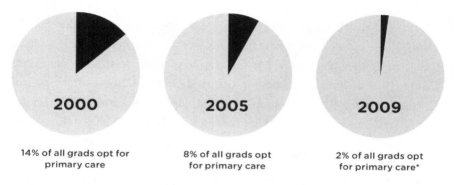

2000

2005

2009

14% of all grads opt for
primary care

8% of all grads opt
for primary care

2% of all grads opt
for primary care*

*Note: Data based on a survey of current students
SOURCE: Association of American Medical Colleges, American Medical Association, *Washington Post*

This discrepancy hints at an even larger one, a disconnect between the aims of medicine—to keep people healthy and maximize our productive life spans—and the practice of medicine. In the United States, this is evident in the declining numbers of primary care doctors, who dropped from 14 percent of all medical school graduates in 2000 to just 2 percent in 2009, even as the need for primary care has increased. It's evident in the growth of specialists, whose ranks have increased accordingly in that same period, a legion trained to step in only after something has already gone wrong. It's evident in the way doctors are compensated, with insurance reimbursements focused on treatments and positive diagnoses, not on prevention and clean bills of health. Even as the medical establishment pays lip service to the idea of preventive medicine and, as we shall see, is adept at identifying new risks and red flags, the actual practice of medicine is firmly rooted in treating symptoms. For the patient, medicine is a lifelong game of "I told you so."

The story is slightly different in the public health world, which is concerned with health at the population level rather than the individual level of clinical medicine. Remember the purpose of the Framingham study, after all: It isn't meant to improve the health of a few thousand citizens of Framingham. It is an effort to understand what their health says about the 300 million other Americans.

That's not to say that the lessons of Framingham don't hold meaning for individuals. Broadly speaking, Framingham has already taught us to avoid too much fat and sugar and to exercise more. And more specifically, the research from Framingham has been turned into calculators that compute what's known as Framingham risk scores. A physician can enter your weight, age, smoking status, diabetes status, and cholesterol level and get a percent risk of your developing cardiovascular disease. And you can do it, too. A quick Google search will turn up a dozen calculators based on Framingham data that churn out a percent risk for everything from atrial fibrillation to stroke. All of these rely on a straightforward formula that combines a person's age, blood cholesterol levels (both HDL, or "good," cholesterol and LDL, or "bad," cholesterol), blood pressure, and a few other variables. Based on various cutoffs, each variable adds one or two points of risk here or, if you're better than average, removes one or two points there.

These calculators have been around for several years, and they've proven useful in getting people to recognize what their personal risks of disease can be. But there's an opportunity to make them even more detailed and specific. After all, considering the multitude of things that go into who you are—your diet, your temperament, your job stress, your commute, your relationship—the idea that your forecast for disease can be based on just four or five factors may seem to rather underestimate your complexity as an individual. It's still several degrees removed from what may or may not be going on in your body. The Framingham study continues to be among the most important sources of data for medical research out there. But no matter how skilled the physician, the actual risk score we get still reflects a distance between our own metrics and abstract science.

The opportunity that a Decision Tree approach offers, then, is to combine into one system the power of population research and the data we draw from ourselves individually. This is the true opportunity presented by personalized, preventive medicine. We need to factor individual information into the equation, to customize the science—science that is powerful, amazing, cutting-edge stuff—to individuals. And we need to deliver the science to people in a way that lets them make sense of it and make use of it. It needs to be information that we can act on and integrate into our lives, information that gives us some control over our health, not information we leave in a pile with all the other advice and warnings we receive.

This is where the tools of self-tracking and self-monitoring become so powerful. Each of us, every day, makes choices and acts in ways that could be quantified, could be broken down into numbers. We have an opportunity to capture this information and enter it into our health equations. These important inputs would make our health care more specific, more precisely about us, rather than about some composite individual from Massachusetts. If the Quantified Self crowd is right, the geeky things they're up to will be filtering down to the rest of us soon (and they are, even now). The tools for self-monitoring are everywhere, and many are remarkably easy to use. The best of these aren't gimmicky gadgets; they offer self-awareness and a way to do it scientifically, rigorously, methodically. To do it with data. To do it with evidence. To do it with numbers.

FOR A FIRST GLIMPSE of what living by numbers looks like today, a fine place to start is at a Kaiser Permanente clinic located on the Hawaiian island of Maui.

Kaiser Permanente is a managed care organization with about 9 million patients across California and nine other states. It's a closed system; once you join Kaiser, you go to Kaiser doctors for all your needs, from primary care to surgery to chronic pain. Though it sounds like the kind of HMO we've come to loathe, Kaiser has long lived by the mantra of "patient care first." It has been a consistent innovator in health care, being among the first health care systems in the country to emphasize preventive care and the first organization of its size to adopt electronic health records. Those records are a boon to efficiency at Kaiser. They allow the organization to e-mail with patients and to avoid prescribing unsafe drug combinations. But the health records also serve as a vast database of insight, allowing the organization to learn from its patients' histories. In other words, it turns Kaiser into a living laboratory with 9 million lab rats.

Kaiser's Maui Lani Clinic is halfway between the Dunes golf course and Kahului Harbor in Maui's biggest city, Wailuku. Maui has the lowest number of doctors per capita in Hawaii, and a higher population of elderly than average. These two factors mean that the Kaiser clinic is more likely to see people after something has already gone wrong.

Accordingly, the clinic has started using what it calls a Panel Support Tool, essentially a computer program that churns out information on the gaps in patients' care *before* they come in to the clinic. The idea is simple: Kaiser took population data from Framingham and the Centers for Disease Control and Prevention and tailored them for its Hawaiian population. Using the electronic health record, in which visits, conditions, medications, and basic information like weight, blood pressure, and cholesterol are logged, the patient's history is compared with best practices on both the national and local levels. An algorithm plugs away in the background, churning through the clinic's patient database. When a patient's data trend line indicates that a red flag may arise ahead—an increasing cholesterol count, say, that is creeping close to the danger zone—then he or she is notified to come in for a visit. A message is also sent to the patient's primary care doctor.

By using the computerized prediction tool to detect what a physician might not yet recognize, Kaiser is pulling every bit of meaning out of a patient's data. What's more, it's engaging the patient in the decision making. The results have been surprising. The Maui clinic has managed to boost the rate of colorectal cancer screening, a notoriously uncomfortable procedure that many people try to avoid, from 31 percent of appropriate patients to 41 percent. Even better, 75 percent of patients at a high risk for heart disease now take aspirin, an effective preventive step, compared to 54 percent previously. Likewise, 74 percent are now on statin therapy, up from 68 percent. The success of Kaiser's tool demonstrates that adding an individual's data into a health calculation can be tremendously effective.

Some other hospitals and health organizations, including the Cleveland Clinic and Scripps Health in San Diego, are pursuing similar patient-centric, data-driven preventive strategies. But until these become the standard rather than the exception, most individuals will have to start living by their numbers on their own.

"Medicine is about to go from analog to digital," says Craig Mundie, Microsoft's chief research and strategy officer and health evangelist. "This means that manual processes [like diagnosis] are moving to a set of automated processes. Of course, medicine, from a business point of view, is resistant to this sort of reengineering. So we wanted to see what Microsoft could do to anticipate these changes and introduce technology that makes it more graceful to move from the old model to a data-driven model."

That's the thinking behind Microsoft's HealthVault service, a new sort of Web-based personal health record. At its most basic, HealthVault is simply a place to assemble and manage our own health records online. This could mean simply loading the data from our doctors' offices and hospitals. But it could also mean a lot more. Microsoft has worked with various manufacturers—companies that make scales, heart-rate monitors, blood pressure cuffs, and so on—to make it possible for users to upload the data from these devices into their health records automatically. The result is constant, real-time data monitoring of all sorts of health inputs.

The way Mundie describes it, these inputs aren't just additive, they're transformative. "Right now, our health is episodic. It's based on what-ever happens in our doctor's office during a visit, or the tests they order. It comes in these chunks. But there's all this ambient information that's also important health information. And if you have continuous health monitoring, you can see trend lines. We can run analytics to create new medicine." What's more, Mundie says, constant tracking of health data can change the way we perceive our health. Right now, that doctor-centric approach starts with one question: What's wrong? But constant tracking, Mundie says, "moves the current negative feedback cycle to an increasingly positive feedback cycle that's data driven. Your health record becomes a platform for invention and improvement."

HealthVault is an illustration of what Mundie calls a "Copernican shift in global health care," where "the patient is moving to the center of the health care universe." Of course Mundie, for obvious reasons, is hoping that HealthVault is the tool we bring with us when we get there (Google has a competing product called Google Health). But, all the same, he's absolutely right that a shift is under way—one that may not be visible in most doctors' offices or hospitals or clinics. There is an opportunity here to think about our health in a new way and to integrate new tools and methods into the fabric of our health.

But perhaps this sounds like a lot of work. And it will be, at least at first. To begin with, we'll have to assert our right to access our own information. How many of us demand a copy of our lab tests when we give up some blood? Or a copy of our x-rays? In order to live by the numbers, we'll have to take charge of our data. We'll have to be vigilant about keeping track of our tracking. And we'll have to deal with numbers.

A lot of numbers.

III.

FOR WOMEN OF A CERTAIN AGE, hormone replacement therapy (HRT) seemed like a godsend in the 1980s and 1990s, when it was widely used as a treatment for menopause. A daily dose of estrogen or a more potent combination of estrogen and progestin (another hormone) seemed to control the mood swings, the hot flashes, and the discomfort that so often come with menopause. It made women feel better and feel younger. What's more, HRT also had the added benefit, it was thought, of reducing the risks of heart disease and osteoporosis. The therapy was recommended to any woman past age 50 who had undergone menopause, and as of July 16, 2002, millions of American women swore by the treatment. It was exactly what modern medicine is supposed to be: a good thing that improves our lives.

And then, all at once, it turned into something bad.

On July 17, 2002, *JAMA*, issued a paper that dramatically contradicted the previous research. A 5-year study called the Women's Health Initiative (WHI), which tracked 8,500 women on HRT and another 8,100 on a placebo, found an alarming correspondence between the

combined estrogen-progestin hormone therapy and increased inci-
dences of heart disease, stroke, and breast cancer. Instead of reducing
women's risk, combination HRT actually seemed to increase it. The
WHI study was supposed to run until 2005, but the results were so
alarming and the therapy apparently so dangerous that the study was
terminated 2½ years early. Women in the study on combination HRT
were told to stop taking it, and the results were quickly compiled and
published in an issue of *JAMA,* one of medicine's most widely read
medical journals.

The *JAMA* article caused a furor. The turnabout on HRT—the miracle that turned out to be a curse—grabbed headlines in the *New York
Times* and the *Wall Street Journal.* The story led the network newscasts.
Jacques Rossouw, MD, the director of the WHI study, put out a statement telling those 6 million women on combined hormone therapy that
they "should have a serious talk with their doctor to see if they should
continue it. . . . Longer term use or use for disease prevention must be
re-evaluated given the multiple adverse effects noted." A *JAMA* editorial
used stronger language: "We recommend that clinicians stop prescribing
this combination for long-term use. . . . The WHI provides an important
health answer for generations of healthy postmenopausal women to
come—do not use estrogen/progestin to prevent chronic disease."

So how did American women react? Within 6 months of the
announcement, about 38 percent of the women had stopped taking the
hormones. By 2004, some 50 percent stopped in response to the WHI
results. Those numbers are okay, but not great—some 2 million women
continue to use combined HRT—but the message was getting through.

But what message, exactly, was it? Even though the WHI specifically implicated only the combined estrogen-progestin therapy, use of
estrogen-only therapy also declined by more than one-third. In the years
following the 2002 announcement, numerous surveys asked women to
explain what they understood the hormone therapy controversy to be
about. Time after time, the consensus was tinged with fear and doubt
rather than clarity and insight. In the technology world, they call this
FUD—short for fear, uncertainty, and doubt. It's not a good thing.

When you're trying to educate people on their health, FUD is just about the worst result you can leave people with.

The problem was that the purpose of HRT changed from one that had clear and widespread benefits to one whose effects were more ambiguous. Not even combination hormone replacement could be considered dangerous for every individual—the WHI found that the increased risk of combined therapy was 19 events per 10,000 person-years, meaning that many women—*most* women, in fact—could use the therapy for years without ever experiencing a negative event. Indeed, most women could use HRT and experience only the benefits of a less uncomfortable menopause. But some people would suffer the side effects, which were severe and often lethal. And there was no way to predict who those few people were, no way to anticipate which individuals would react poorly. So on a population level, it was too dangerous to recommend to anybody. This gap between the population implications and the implications for any one individual explains the confusing recommendation from the WHI director to have a "serious talk" rather than his clearly saying "*Stop.*"

Health economists call this difference between obviously beneficial treatments and marginally beneficial ones a distinction between "effective" treatments and "preference-sensitive" treatments. Effective treatments are those whose benefits far outweigh their harms, and the goal of medicine should be to disseminate them wide and far. That's what HRT was thought to be. In preference-sensitive treatments, though, the trade-offs are subtler, and thus more personal. In these cases, it's up to each patient to educate herself and come to an informed decision. That's what HRT became.

The history of medical science starts with effective treatments—surgery, vaccines, and antibiotics—whose benefits clearly outweighed their detriments. But as with other sciences, bold innovations in medicine come less often these days; discoveries increasingly result from a process of winnowing out smaller, more incremental innovations. And with these discoveries, the benefits are less sweeping and more precise. This precision is largely a good thing—as patients, we want to know in greater detail what risks a treatment poses to whom, based on data. We want to know what *our* risks are; we want a treatment that works for *us*. But there is a trade-off, in that the risks and benefits are not always so easily weighed. *Risk,* after all, is another word for "chance," and chance means there's always a possibility that something may or may not happen, whatever the odds may be.

This is the challenge we all face today, whenever we go to the doctor's office. And it's a challenge that will only grow more pronounced as medical science develops ever-finer gradations of risk. And it's one we ourselves will have to face up to more often, as Craig Mundie's Copernican shift takes place and we become the stewards of our own health. The opportunity of choice will be our burden.

UNDERSTANDING OUR HEALTH RISKS—part of what is often called health literacy—isn't simply a matter of having information. We don't lack statistics. We lack a system to make sense of them. "There are a lot of studies that supposedly show how stupid people are," says Lisa Schwartz, MD, a physician and information expert at the Dartmouth Institute for Health Policy and Clinical Practice in Lebanon, New Hampshire. "But information is usually presented in a way that's harder than it has to be. People already have skills to understand this information; they're skills they're using in other areas of their lives—shopping, driving."

Dr. Schwartz and her husband, Steven Woloshin, MD (also a physician at the Dartmouth Institute), have made a mission of advocating for the clear, comprehensible presentation of health information. Among their other efforts, they've created what they call a Drug Facts box—a simple table designed to appear on drug labels that's an antidote to the indecipherable blather we now get on those labels and in drug advertising. Instead of all that unintelligible jargon and fine print, Dr. Schwartz's and Dr. Woloshin's label makes a few clear statements. What is this drug for? Who is it for? Who shouldn't take it? And then it gets to the particulars: How well does the drug meet its purpose? The Drug Facts box distills the results of the clinical trials a drug must go through for Food and Drug Administration (FDA) approval into some clear factual points: What difference did the drug make for the intended condition compared

A Better Way to Label Drugs

A Drug Facts box can turn the mystifying fine print of drug advertisements into clear, useful information.

DRUG FACTS
TAMOXIFEN (Nolvadex)

What is this drug for?
To reduce the chance of getting breast cancer

Who might consider taking it?
Women at high risk of getting breast cancer (1.7% or higher risk over 5 years). You can calculate your breast cancer risk at http://bcra.nci.nih.gov/btc.

Who should not take it?
Women who are pregnant or breastfeeding

Recommended testing:
Have a yearly checkup that includes a gynecological examination and blood tests

Other things to consider doing:
No other medicines are approved to reduce breast cancer risk for women who have not had breast cancer.

TAMOXIFEN STUDY FINDINGS TABLE

13,000 women at high risk of getting breast cancer were given TAMOXIFEN or a sugar pill for 6 years. Here's what happened:

What difference did TAMOXIFEN make?	Women given a sugar pill	Women given TAMOXIFEN (20 mg a day)
How did TAMOXIFEN help?		
Fewer women got invasive breast cancer	3.3%	1.7%
(1.6% fewer due to drug)		
No difference in death from breast cancer	About 0.09% in both groups	
What were TAMOXIFEN's side effects?		
Life-threatening side effects		
More women had a blood clot in their leg or lungs	0.5%	1.0%
(additional 0.5% due to drug)		
More women got invasive uterine cancer	0.5%	1.1%
(additional 0.6% due to drug)		
Symptom side effects		
More women had hot flashes	68%	80%
(additional 12% due to drug)		
More women had vaginal discharge	35%	55%
(additional 20% due to drug)		
More women had cataracts needing surgery	1.5%	2.3%
(additional 0.8% due to drug)		
Bottom line		
No difference in deaths from all causes combined	About 1.2% in both groups	

How long has the drug been in use?
Tamoxifen was first approved by the FDA in 1992 for the treatment of breast cancer. It was approved for preventing breast cancer in 1998. Since the drug has been used by large numbers of people over a longer time, the emergence of rare but serious side effects is less likely than for new drugs.

with a placebo, and how many people experienced side effects with it compared with a placebo?

The Drug Facts box is modeled on the Nutrition Facts label that's now required on nearly all packaged food products in the United States. "It's crazy that we require our Cocoa Krispies to have standardized labels, but not drugs that have serious side effects," Dr. Schwartz suggests. As of this writing, the FDA is considering a recommendation to require the Drug Facts box on pharmaceutical labels.

And the box works. In an experiment, Dr. Schwartz and Dr. Woloshin tested the Drug Facts box against ordinary drug ads to see whether people could correctly parse the information and understand how risky a drug is. They sent two different sets of ads to two groups of consumers. One group received ads for Amcid and Maxtor, two heartburn treatments, with the usual disclosures and fine print (the ads were real, but the names of the drugs and their manufacturers had been changed). The other group received the same ads, but the pharmaceutical companies' disclosure statements were replaced with Drug Facts boxes that the researchers had created using data from the clinical trials performed to secure FDA approval. Both groups were asked to imagine that they had heartburn and then to choose the drug that they thought would be more effective.

In truth, Maxtor was the more effective drug, so it would be the "right" answer. But the group that looked at the standard ads decided otherwise: 70 percent of them chose Amcid, the "wrong" drug for their condition, based on the evidence. Something about the ads caused most of them to make the wrong choice. Among the group looking at the Drug Facts box, though, the numbers were exactly reversed: 70 percent correctly chose Maxtor as the better drug. What's more, the Drug Facts box group was better informed about the drugs' side effects: 51 percent answered correctly about the possible side effects, compared to just 16 percent among the group looking at the ordinary ads.

The results were vindicating, says Dr. Schwartz, demonstrating not just how well the Drug Facts box works, but also that ordinary people can navigate through difficult statistics if they're given the right tools. "This is hard information. It meant sorting out two tables of numbers about side effects and benefits. And they had to read it, to synthesize it.

And most of them did. We were really impressed that people did so well. People are smarter than we give them credit for."

That's especially important considering the volume of health information people are expected to navigate now—and how much more they're going to have to comprehend soon enough. There are data about risks for disease, about drugs, and about the side effects of drugs. There are screening statistics to navigate, treatments to weigh against each other. And now genetics is entering the picture as well. For Dr. Schwartz, putting individuals in charge of so many health decisions means we need to think hard about how we deliver that information. We need to put a priority on making information something that benefits people rather than baffles them.

Because there's always the alternative: Stay in the dark, don't seek access to information, and rely on the doctor to sort it out. That, after all, is how it has worked for a long time. Willful ignorance is always an option—but it's not the best option. "People face an up-front decision," Dr. Schwartz says. "Do you want to go down this path? Do you want to understand how big the risks you face are, the risks and benefits of a treatment? Do you really want to go down the medical path of monitoring and treatment? It's important that we make that first decision in a conscious way. Because this information can be powerful; it can help people make good decisions. People want control, and this can help create that. But we need to help people not overreact to uncertain information. Because there will always be uncertainty."

IV.

IN THE 1920S, the Western Electric Company ran an experiment. Company managers wanted to test whether brighter or dimmer lighting in their Hawthorne Works factory in Chicago had any influence over their workers' productivity. So every few hours, the factory lights were adjusted, sometimes up, sometimes down. Then they measured whether the factory workers made more relays or fewer.

As it turned out, the workers increased their output *regardless* of whether the lights were brightened or dimmed. A change in the lighting, it seemed, served as a cue to the employees that they were under observation. And so they picked up the pace. This phenomenon became known as the Hawthorne effect, which holds that simply watching people can change their behavior.

As it turns out, the story may be too good to be true. In 2009, Steven Levitt, the economist and coauthor of *Freakonomics,* and another University of Chicago economist got access to the original data. It seems that no valid measurement was done to prove an effect at the Hawthorne Works. But regardless of the veracity of that original story, the effect itself seems to be a real phenomenon that has since been documented many times under more rigorous circumstances. And the Hawthorne effect has corollaries in other sciences as well. The Heisenberg uncertainty principle in physics, the placebo effect in pharmacology, and selection bias in epidemiology all describe a similar phenomenon: When something is under observation, particularly in an experiment, the behavior of that something can change, particularly among human beings.

Medical research, and population research in particular, is especially vulnerable to the Hawthorne effect. If people are participating in a study on, say, whether a certain drug lowers blood pressure, there's always the chance that there is some influence, perhaps impossible to measure, being wielded by the experiment itself. Most experiments are designed to take some account of this possibility. The very idea of a double-blind experiment is to make both the scientist and the subject unaware of who is taking the real medicine and who is getting the sugar pill. But there's no escaping the fact that the structure of the test itself—the fact that people have been asked to participate in a study and that they often know what the purpose of the study is—can play a role in how somebody feels and behaves. Science, in this way, will always be an imperfect thing.

The Hawthorne effect has been measured in research on high blood pressure, diabetes, and other conditions that require constant self-monitoring. In most of these studies, the effect has typically been seen as a negative, something that distorts the purity of the study. But recently, the idea has been turned around: Maybe the Hawthorne effect is not necessarily a bad thing. Maybe it can be put to work on our behalf. A

2006 study in a German hospital found that simply telling staff that their "hygienic performance" was being monitored improved hand washing by 55 percent—an insight that's particularly relevant to hospitals, considering the growing risk of hospital-acquired infections.

And then there's a 2002 study that tried to see whether the Hawthorne effect would have any impact on getting teenagers to brush their teeth. The idea here wasn't just to measure the Hawthorne effect, it was to exploit it, to deliberately *trick* kids into having better habits.

The experiment started at a Kansas City orthodontic clinic. Using patients' records, the researchers identified 40 adolescent patients with especially poor dental hygiene. Half of them weren't told they would be monitored (all patients at the clinic had previously signed a catchall consent form that agreed to the standard collection of patient information); this would be the control group, whose members would be observed but wouldn't know it. Those in the other half were the guinea pigs: They would be observed and they'd *know* they were being observed.

It all seemed very serious. The 20 in the experimental group were asked to join an experiment to test the effectiveness of a new orthodontic toothpaste. They'd have to brush their teeth twice a day for 2 minutes at a spell. They were given 2-minute timers to put on their sinks and asked to use them every time they brushed in order to ensure that they met the full duration. And then they were sent home with special tubes of toothpaste marked with their patient numbers and labeled "Experimental." This was special stuff, so they were asked to return any unused toothpaste after 6 months.

What was this new, high-tech, super-experimental toothpaste? Just ordinary Crest with fluoride.

After 3 months, the subjects came back for checkups. Digital photographs were taken, and a computer calculated their plaque scores (the ratio of plaque to the total tooth surface, a standard measure of dental hygiene). At the start of the experiment, the control and experimental groups had roughly the same plaque scores, about 70 percent. But after just 12 weeks, the subjects using the "Experimental" toothpaste had reduced their plaque levels to 54 percent. The control group, meanwhile, had gotten a little lazier, with their plaque scores rising to 78 percent.

After 6 months, the trend lines widened even more: The experimental group had plaque scores of 52 percent while the control set rose to 79 percent. Since the special toothpaste was ordinary Crest, and since all the patients had access to the same information and all had been told to brush their teeth, there was nothing to explain the difference—except the fact that half of the kids knew they were being monitored while the other half did not. Outfitted with nothing more than a timer and a more conscious sense of what they were doing, the kids in the experiment improved their behavior and had better teeth to show for it.

What should we make of the Hawthorne effect, other than that it reflects a curious bit of human psychology? Just this: Perhaps the Hawthorne effect is something we can turn to our advantage consciously, just as it was turned to the advantage of those teenagers unconsciously. The idea of living by numbers is really to be aware of what we're doing, to engage with health information, including those metrics that we ourselves are generating, in positive, healthful ways. The objective of using Decision Tree thinking is really to put the Hawthorne effect, and any other tools, to work for us. Simply paying attention to our health, thinking about it explicitly as something we are mindful of, may already be putting us on a better track.

This has been demonstrated, somewhat remarkably, in data gathered by the National Weight Control Registry, a database of more than 5,000 individuals who have lost a significant amount of weight and managed to keep it off. Since 1994, the registry has conducted surveys of these successful losers in the hope of identifying effective strategies for sustained weight loss. Among the most powerful factors in success, the study has found, is the simple act of stepping on a scale. Eighty percent of registry participants weigh themselves at least once a week, and more than a third weigh themselves daily. And when daily scale-steppers dropped off in their monitoring, they began to eat more, and sure enough they started to gain weight back. Paying attention matters.

What works for weight loss likely works in other health matters as well. Using the tools of self-monitoring, we can put the Hawthorne effect into action. The combination could lead to that greater sense of control that the Whitehall study found to be so essential. By tracking our data and charting our progress toward better health, we are really turning ourselves into experiments. And after all, what's a more fascinating, more important subject for sustained examination than ourselves?

WALKING THROUGH SHOPPER'S WORLD in Framingham, it's hard not to wonder whether being the birthplace of risk-based medicine has made Framingham a better-informed, healthier town. On the one hand, the people look normal enough—for good and for bad. Even on a cold and rainy afternoon, a few folks huddle outside the mall entrance smoking cigarettes. And for all the people headed to the linens store, there are plenty of others—many overweight or obese—making their way to the bar and grill.

On the other hand, though, some study participants hint at something that might be the Hawthorne effect at work. "Filling out that sheet made me think about what I was eating, how much I was exercising," one study participant confessed. "I learned to cook differently, and our kids grew up eating differently. They're very aware of good nutrition and the importance of exercise."

In essence, this is the opportunity a Decision Tree offers. We don't need to be enrolled in a study conducted by the National Institutes of Health or have dozens of doctors monitoring us. And it doesn't mean we need to obsess over every last metric that we can record about ourselves. But by looking to the numbers—whether from Framingham or Whitehall or our own selves—we can turn their meaning into better decisions. We can take control of our destinies.

Toxic Knowledge

How DNA Got to Be So Scary,
and Why It Shouldn't Be

I.

TERI SMIEJA HAD A CHOICE TO MAKE. A mother of two living in the small town of Ridgecrest, California, Teri learned in February 2009 that she has a much higher risk of developing breast and ovarian cancers than the typical American woman. And now she needed to figure out what to do about it.

It had actually happened very fast. In late 2008, her aunt had gone on a trip to Israel. When she came back to the States, she explained to Teri that Ashkenazi Jews like themselves were more likely to have mutations in two genes known as *BRCA1* and *BRCA2*. Those mutations put women at a much higher risk for breast or ovarian cancer—60 percent or higher (the average American female has about a 12 percent risk). For Teri, who didn't really identify as Jewish, this was all brand-new. "I had never heard of Ashkenazi anything before," she says, let alone heard of *BRCA* genes. But she did know that ovarian cancer ran in her family— her grandmother had had it, her mother has it, her aunt had it. "I always figured I had a higher chance of getting cancer," she says, but she hadn't known there was a way to measure that risk.

So in December 2008, Teri took a test, and, 3 months and one botched lab result later, she found out the results: She was positive for the *BRCA1* mutation. The question now was what to do next. "I had this paper in my hand that said I have up to an 87 percent risk of getting cancer by age 70. And of course I started crying; I was really upset. But then it hit me: It didn't say I *had* cancer; it said I *could get* cancer. So I said to myself, stop feeling sorry for yourself. This is good news. I can do something about this."

About 5 to 10 percent of breast cancers are thought to be inherited, most of them through a *BRCA1* or *BRCA2* mutation (a *BRCA2* mutation raises the lifetime risk of breast cancer to about 60 percent). The mutations are often found in women of Ashkenazi Jewish descent, as in Teri's case, but they also turn up among people of other ethnicities. Because estrogen promotes cell division in women, it's often recommended that women with an increased risk have their ovaries and uteruses removed, since the ovaries produce most of the estrogen in the female body. As far as these sorts of procedures go, oophorectomy with hysterectomy is relatively low impact; the procedure can be performed laparoscopically in about 45 minutes. It's often an outpatient procedure, although a woman without ovaries undergoes premature menopause. Many women with a high risk also opt for a preemptive mastectomy, because estrogen receptors in the breasts make them the prime targets of the cancer. A mastectomy is a more traumatic procedure, both in terms of recovering from the wounds and for social and psychological reasons. A woman seeking to absolutely minimize her chances of developing cancer would undergo both procedures.

For women like Teri, the prospect of having both procedures is a quandary of profound implications, a decision that's incredibly difficult to navigate. In a term that reflects the genetic age we live in, these women are known as previvors—they don't have a cancer yet. But they surely have something.

After spending a lot of time on the Internet and visiting a genetic counselor ("They said I did it wrong. I was supposed to go to the counselor first," she recalls), Teri had decided that she was definitely doing the oophorectomy and hysterectomy. "It cuts your risk of breast cancer

Teri Smieja's Decision Tree

Teri knew that ovarian cancer ran in her family, but it wasn't until her aunt told her about *BRCA* mutations that she realized she could take a test to learn her risk. That one decision led to several more.

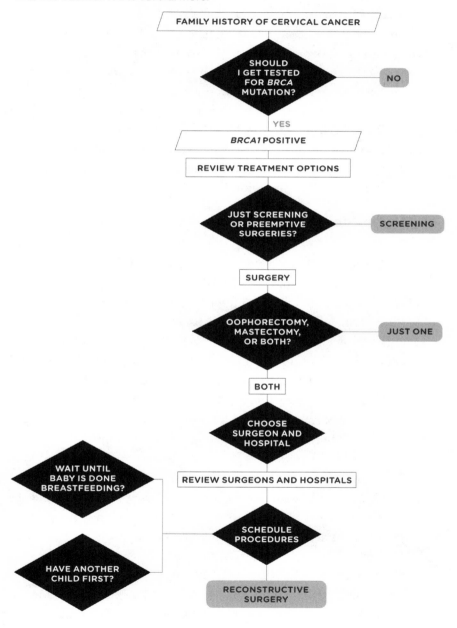

FAMILY HISTORY OF CERVICAL CANCER

SHOULD I GET TESTED FOR *BRCA* MUTATION? — NO

YES

BRCA1 POSITIVE

REVIEW TREATMENT OPTIONS

JUST SCREENING OR PREEMPTIVE SURGERIES? — SCREENING

SURGERY

OOPHORECTOMY, MASTECTOMY, OR BOTH? — JUST ONE

BOTH

CHOOSE SURGEON AND HOSPITAL

WAIT UNTIL BABY IS DONE BREASTFEEDING?

REVIEW SURGEONS AND HOSPITALS

HAVE ANOTHER CHILD FIRST?

SCHEDULE PROCEDURES

RECONSTRUCTIVE SURGERY

by about half," she says. She had the procedure in early October 2009, barely 6 months after learning of her risk.

And she's certain—almost certain—that she's going to have the preemptive double mastectomy (also known as a prophylactic bilateral mastectomy, or PBM) as well. The thing is, she says, "I'm usually really bad with decisions. Ask me 'Where do you want to eat?' and I'll say, 'I don't know, you choose!' So deciding this has been the hardest part. And I'm 90 percent a yes on the PBM. Every once in a while I'll have a tremor and think I shouldn't, but the majority of me says yes. This is what I need to do. I need to be around for my kids. I am not my ovaries. I am not my breasts. So now it's just the process. I have to decide where to get the procedure done, I have to schedule doctors. I still have a long battle ahead, but I think I'm done with that decision."

I GREW UP IN MINNEAPOLIS in the 1970s, where I attended a Catholic grade school. True to the stereotype, there was no lack of large broods of seven, eight, or nine kids—Kellys and Costellos and Kedrowskis (with a mere four children in our family, the Goetzes ranked as a smallish clan). Among so many big families, there were a couple of schoolmates who had a sister or brother with Down syndrome. This wasn't common, certainly, but it wasn't exactly uncommon. It seemed like simple statistics, the laws of chance on display in real life.

Nearly 40 years later, it seems uncommon indeed to see a child with Down syndrome. And the statistics bear this observation out: The number of children born with Down syndrome has fallen by about 15 to 20 percent since the mid-1980s in the United States, the United Kingdom, Australia, and much of Europe. That's exactly the opposite direction the demographic trends would imply, given our aging population and the fact that women are choosing to have children later in life. Going by those trends, the number of Down syndrome births should have *increased* by 30 percent or more. So what happened?

A genetic test.

In the late 1970s, a prenatal test called amniocentesis was introduced that checks for the chromosomal abnormality that causes Down syndrome. In amniocentesis, a small amount of amniotic fluid is extracted from the uterus of the expectant mother; the fluid is then used to make an image of the fetus's 23 pairs of chromosomes. An extra chromosome at the 21st position indicates the birth defect we call Down syndrome. Studies have found that among American mothers who undergo amnio (or one of several newer tests for prenatal defects) and receive a positive result, about 90 percent decide to terminate the pregnancy. The numbers are similar in Europe and Australia.

The upshot of all this testing is that there are simply fewer children coming into the world with Down syndrome. And the numbers are likely to fall even further and even faster: Since 2007, the American College of Obstetricians and Gynecologists has recommended that *all* women be offered prenatal screening for Down syndrome (previously the test was only recommended for women more than 35 years old).

The test for Down syndrome is just one of several genetic tests that have become a routine part of pregnancy for American women. Today,

Genetic Tests At or Before Birth

Genetic testing is already standard practice in prenatal care and pediatrics. Here's a rundown of routine tests.

PRENATAL
- Amniocentesis
- Chorionic villus sampling (CVS)
- Down syndrome
- Hemoglobinopathies
- Hemophilia A
- Alpha- and beta-thalassemia
- Polycystic kidney disease (adult type)
- Sickle cell anemia
- Fragile X syndrome
- Cystic fibrosis
- Congenital adrenal hyperplasia
- Duchenne muscular dystrophy
- Ashkenazi Jewish Panel (including Tay-Sachs and eight other conditions)

NEWBORN
- Cystic fibrosis
- Primary congenital hypothyroidism (and variant)
- MS/MS screening
- Amino acid disorders (17 other conditions)
- Organic acid disorders (17 other conditions)
- Fatty acid oxidation disorders (11 other conditions)
- Hemoglobin disorders (more than two dozen others)

SOURCES: American College of Medical Genetics, Merck, California Department of Health Services, National Newborn Screening and Genetics Resource Center

more than half of mothers undergo some form of genetic testing, including tests for Down syndrome, neural tube defects, trisomy 18, and cystic fibrosis. These tests are having a radical impact on the appearance of these diseases in society. A recent study in the *Journal of Pediatrics* found that cases of cystic fibrosis have declined by 30 percent in the Brittany area of France since 1990. Ninety-three percent of women who had a positive test for cystic fibrosis opted to end the pregnancy.

These are grave choices—big, weighty decisions based on heartfelt values and beliefs. The opportunity to intervene and change the course of a life, even by choosing to end a pregnancy, is a profound and deeply personal matter. Indeed, the above numbers are hard for researchers to come by, because the statistics and the decisions they represent are so closely protected by hospitals.

For most people, prenatal screening is our first brush with genetics. It's where this abstract science suddenly gets very personal, and it comes laced with portent and drama. Typically, we don't even discuss the results with a physician. Instead, a genetic counselor—someone specially trained to deliver this weighty information—handles the job, helping us navigate the issues, answering the questions that will bring us to a decision.

Increasingly, life brings other genetic tests as well. Just as breast cancer can be caused by a *BRCA1* or *BRCA2* mutation, so too is Huntington's disease (an untreatable neurological disorder that starts its inexorable mental deterioration in the prime of life, in the thirties and forties) caused by genetics, as are fragile X syndrome (an inherited class of conditions that can resemble mental retardation or autism) and muscular dystrophy (a disease characterized by progressive and irreversible muscle weakness). These are dire diseases fraught with anxiety and often, since treating genetic conditions can be so difficult, despair.

There are valid genetic tests for nearly 2,000 conditions, according to the list at GeneTests (www.ncbi.nlm.nih.gov/sites/GeneTests), a catalog funded by the National Institutes of Health. For most of these tests, the stakes are about as high as they come in contemporary life. A positive test equals either disease or a dramatically high probability of developing disease, and that information often changes the courses of lives.

Pregnancies are terminated, wills are drawn up, marriages are ended, major surgeries are undertaken. The stakes are so serious that bioethicists have a term for the information the tests deliver: "Toxic knowledge" they call it, because the results can be so significant as to be dangerous.

"I'm a card-carrying geneticist," says Harry Ostrer, MD, the head of the Human Genetics Program in the department of pediatrics at the New York University School of Medicine. "And I think there should be limits for certain types of genetic tests. Learning the results could be harmful to people when there is no treatment. Also I think people are going to learn about personal risks that they aren't necessarily prepared to hear. You go to the doctor and all of a sudden he's telling you about your risk for this or that. You could say, 'Gee, I was here for a blood test and now you're telling me about increased risk for Parkinson's disease?' That to me is the dark side of genetic testing."

For years, the overwhelming concern about genetic information has been that it will be used against us, that our insurance companies will deny us health care or our employers will fire us because of our genes. That fear became less pressing in 2008, when President George W. Bush signed the Genetic Information Nondiscrimination Act, or GINA, which prohibits employers and health insurers from discriminating based on DNA. But the law itself is suffused with fear about the uncertain power of genetic information (indeed, the fact that GINA was written into the civil rights code, alongside the Voting Rights Act and the 19th Amendment, says something about how seriously we take the fears about genetic information).

But is genetic information really so toxic? Is knowledge about our genomes so peculiar, such a disconcerting glimpse through the gauze of day-to-day life and into the future beyond, that it's dangerous, even poisonous?

ONE OF THE CENTRAL ARGUMENTS of this book is that the answer is no. This notion that genetic information, or indeed any health information, can somehow be dangerous—that knowledge itself is somehow destructive, that individuals must be protected from knowing about themselves—is a dated and indeed *more* dangerous notion. I'm not suggesting that genetics isn't serious business. There are many reasons to be frightened of a genetic test, just as there is reason to be frightened about the results of a biopsy or an MRI. These tests all tell us something we didn't know, and that information may not be what we might wish. But the tone of the conversation about DNA today is outdated, akin to the way doctors not too long ago wouldn't tell their patients about cancer diagnoses or would hedge on their chances for survival. There's nothing intrinsic to genetic information, in and of itself, that makes it different from other information about our health. And there's certainly nothing in it that's *inherently* destructive, over and above other sorts of information. Genetic tests can be powerful and they can be life altering. But if we've learned to fear that knowledge, we've learned the wrong lesson about genetics.

What's happened with genetics is a sort of bioethical hiccup: Our social understanding of the science is locked into an anachronistic conception of that science. And while the science has evolved, revealing the more nuanced and less deterministic role of genetics, the popular perception that genetic information is to be feared has not. The idea that genes equal destiny, that genetic information is so potent that it is toxic, is a legacy of limited scientific understanding.

There was a time, 20 years back, when all genetic information carried dire consequences, because the only tests available were for dire genetic conditions like Down syndrome or Huntington's disease, for which there were usually few or no treatments. *Any* genetic knowledge was dangerous because *all* genetic knowledge was dangerous. But as the science has improved and our understanding of genetics has increased, the information genetics communicates is increasingly less definitive, less than black-and-white. It's no longer all about absolutes and much more about possibilities. It turns out that, in most cases, our genes aren't our fate—for the most part, they don't predetermine our path, they only influence it. That makes genetics more complicated and more difficult to understand, but that is by and large a good thing, more beneficial than destructive.

After all, another name for genetics is simply *family history*. When we think back to what our grandparents died of and what health issues our parents may be struggling with, that's thinking about genetics. Family histories are a great opportunity for acting early on our health, for spotting possible patterns that might be red flags for our own futures. The US surgeon general's office has put together a Web site—www.hhs.gov/family history—that helps people construct a thorough family health history, flushing out possible genetic risks for disease along the way. If we're lucky, we'll know enough about what ailments our great-grandparents and great-aunts and -uncles and other relatives have suffered from to make such tools useful. It's not perfect science, but family history is a form of layman's genetics in that we can troll it for clues to what we may be predisposed toward. Our family trees are natural components of our Decision Trees.

The difference is that now, with genetic tests, we can get a more precise understanding of how our predispositions work and where they come from. We can get a peek at just what stuff in ourselves may come from our predecessors, what risks we've inherited, and what risks we may pass along. And by understanding which way our genes may point, we can take actions that will keep us from heading down the wrong paths.

In contrast to the black-and-white reality of a test for Down syndrome, the new frontier of genetics research doesn't typically lead us to life-altering decisions. Most of what we're learning—and need to learn more about—are the nuances, the small and even subtle influences that genetics has on our health. We may have genetic factors that increase our risk of heart disease, so we decide not to smoke that cigar, or perhaps we're genetically more likely to retain fat cells, so we start to follow a healthful diet *before* we begin to put on extra weight. Even a test that shows a condition like a mutation in the *BRCA1* gene, which carries as much as a 60 percent lifetime risk of breast cancer, doesn't necessarily put the recipient in as dire a circumstance today as might've been the case a decade ago. Yes, there are new treatments and new drugs that can improve survival. But even more dramatically, there are new ways of parsing this information, of digesting it, of factoring it into a decision process—a Decision Tree—that can greatly reduce the fog and fear such a test result may have once induced.

This isn't to suggest that this information won't create all sorts of questions, including specific ones that are sometimes uncomfortable. You may learn that you have a genetic risk of developing colon cancer. Should you give up eating meat? If you have a genetic risk of heart disease, should you quit your stressful job and move into a less taxing profession? If you have a *BRCA2* mutation for breast cancer, should you tell your sister that she might face a similar risk? And after you've tested your newborn for various diseases and gotten her vaccinated, why not get a scan of her DNA to see if she should live her life in specific ways, avoiding certain activities or diets, say, or taking up certain sports? (Such tests already exist: Atlas Sports Genetics offers a $149 test for the *ACTN3* gene that has been linked to predispositions for speed or endurance sports.) Each of these decisions carries serious repercussions, some of which cannot be undone. And each will exact an emotional toll.

The purpose of a Decision Tree is precisely this: to offer a strategy for considering new information in a thorough, systematic manner that allows us to make the most of the information, to exploit it rather than be cowed by it. This is where we can learn from Teri Smieja's example. As she learned with her *BRCA1* status, genetic tests can be an opportunity for us to use more information to make earlier choices to avoid worse ones later. Genetic knowledge can create opportunities for decisions, not dilemmas.

Genetic factors, indeed, are on just the first branches of our Decision Trees, parts of a decision process that should lead us to think more often about our long-term health goals. If the core principles behind a Decision Tree are to look early, gather the data, and be open, then genetics embodies all of these. It is the earliest source of information we can gather about ourselves (being available even before birth), and it is data, through and through. And it offers the opportunity for openness, because we can share our genetic profiles with family members, friends, and even strangers on mutual voyages of discovery. Genetics isn't the be-all and end-all of our health choices, but it can be an especially revealing and early window into them.

The problem with treating all genetic information as toxic is that it restricts our opportunity to engage with our DNA, to learn from it, and, perhaps, to improve our lives by that engagement. So the good news is that genetics isn't life or death. But the bad news is that genetics can be more complicated than life or death.

II.

WHEN GREGOR MENDEL BEGAN GROWING PEAS in his abbey's garden in the 1850s, he was just a simple monk curious about the differences among the plants. A member of the Augustinian order, an especially studious sect, Mendel took to his garden experiments with characteristic discipline and rigor. He grew some peas with green seeds and others with yellow ones, some with pink flowers and others with white, some with round seedpods and others with wrinkled pods, and so on—at least 10,000 plants in all. And he took rigorous notes, documenting the traits of every plant and every generation of plants. After half a dozen years in his garden, Mendel had established the principles of genetic inheritance, identifying some traits as dominant and others as recessive.

A hundred and fifty years later, what Mendel learned in his garden remains the cornerstone of genetics. We now understand his traits to be the results of genes, and genes to be sections of DNA—a strand made up of four proteins, or nucleotides, called adenine, cytosine, thymine, and guanine, or ACTG. These four nucleotides line up in pairs in a ladder of 6 billion pairs to compose the genomic code.

Code is very much the right word here; the ACTG of our genome spins out along this 6 billion–pair sequence like a computer program, but one with slight variations from person to person. Each ACTG molecule lines up along a ladder, matched to another ACTG molecule (As usually match up with Ts, and Cs with Gs, but there are exceptions). This ladder, or double helix, as the discoverers of DNA, James Watson, PhD, and Francis Crick, PhD, called it, comes in 23 sections called chromosomes. Within these chromosomes, certain sections of ACTG have specific functions and roles; these sections are what are known as genes. When people say you have a gene for this or a gene for that, technically, this is what they're referring to.

Since 1983, when the gene associated with Huntington's disease was first linked to a particular chromosome, most genetic discoveries have been like those Mendel made with his peas: They have focused on traits associated with single genes. These so-called monogenic conditions—diseases like hemochromatosis (in which the body absorbs too much iron) or Tay-Sachs disease (a neurological disease)—were the easiest to research because the associations are pretty much binary. If you have the genetic mutation, you're almost certain to develop the disease. That makes them easy to test for, too. Careful testing for Tay-Sachs disease among Ashkenazi Jews, for instance, has led to a 90 percent reduction in the disease in the United States and Canada.

But genes, per se, are a somewhat antiquated conception of how our DNA works. As genetic research has progressed, the idea that most diseases will have a clearly defined, single genetic component—what's known as the common disease–common gene hypothesis—has turned out to be mostly wishful thinking. In fact, the more than 2,000 or so conditions that are currently tested for—nearly all monogenic in origin—represent about 5 percent of the disease burden in developed countries, meaning that for 95 percent of that burden, something more complicated is going on.

The code of our DNA doesn't just engage in big units of genes; it also works at the single base pair. If a GAG sequence in the 11th chromosome is normal, for instance, a one-letter slip to a GTG sequence could trigger sickle-cell anemia. This is what's known as a single nucleotide polymorphism, or SNP—a scientific term that simply means a variation in a single base pair.

What's more, most of the diseases we worry about today develop from subtle interplay between the environment and *several* SNPs. They are said to be polygenic or multigenic, not monogenic, diseases. And these conditions, which include the more common chronic conditions that currently impact society (heart disease, cancer, obesity, and so on),

Assessing Risk and Heritability

The pervasiveness of a disease in society does not necessarily correlate to its genetic influence, or heritability. While some prevalent conditions like type 2 diabetes are characterized by a relatively low heritability, less common diagnoses like Huntington's are caused entirely by genetics.

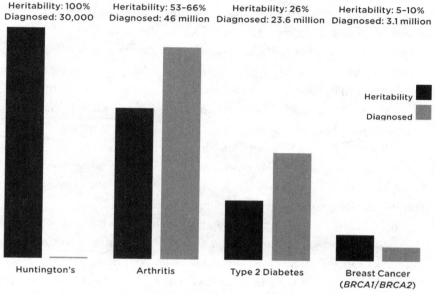

Heritability: 100%
Diagnosed: 30,000

Heritability: 53–66%
Diagnosed: 46 million

Heritability: 26%
Diagnosed: 23.6 million

Heritability: 5–10%
Diagnosed: 3.1 million

Heritability

Diagnosed

Huntington's   Arthritis   Type 2 Diabetes   Breast Cancer
                                                                    (*BRCA1/BRCA2*)

SOURCES: National Institutes of Health, Huntington's Disease Society of America, American Cancer Society, National Cancer Institute, Centers for Disease Control and Prevention, 23andMe

are far harder to match up with their genetic precursors. And doing so requires a greater understanding of the particulars of our genetic codes.

Science is exploring this structure for meaning at several levels. Some geneticists are still hard at work looking at big chunks of DNA for big influences on health and disease. These monogenic conditions, they feel, are the ones that are most clearly associated with genetics, and, given the state of technology, that's where genetic research is most likely to make clear, strong findings. It's still intensely complicated, needle-in-a-haystack work, mind you, but at least the haystacks are a little smaller and the needles a little more obvious.

Other scientists, meanwhile, have taken their test tubes and headed out into the hay fields, looking for the stray signal that may point to a genetic factor in a more common disease. This is the work that extends across the entire genome. Their hope is that they can start to piece together the smaller influences that happen here or there, single-letter variation by single-letter variation, and understand the combinations and relationships that create higher risks for the conditions that affect large numbers of people—heart disease, diabetes, and so forth. (Scientists make the confusing distinction here that "genetics" works at the gene level and "genomics" works across the genome, but for the purposes of this book, both terms refer to the same collective science and are used interchangeably.) For these researchers, the main challenge is establishing which SNPs—or which constellations of SNPs—affect which conditions. At first, this work seemed like it was going to be fairly straightforward, like there would be clear variants that contributed significant—but not absolute—risks for disease.

As the research comes in, though, it's proving that the common disease–common variant hypothesis may also be a bit too wishful. The complexity of the project is unavoidable. It lays out like a matrix: thousands of diseases, billions of genetic variations, untold environmental influences, all combining to create our health. In short, what once looked like a simple explanation for how we turn out is becoming ever more intricate.

So this, in vastly oversimplified form, is the state of genetics 10 years into the 21st century. It's important to be mindful of time here, because our understanding of genetics is changing incredibly fast. Just as chemistry evolved from 4 elements in ancient Greece to 117 today, and physics moved from Newtonian laws to Einstein and quantum complexity, so too has it been with genetics—the more we learn, the more complicated things get.

If nothing else, though, this level of complexity means that the idea that genetic information is toxic information is decidedly outmoded. In most circumstances, there is nothing definitive about genetics; our DNA is *not* our destiny. Genetic information now is more likely to be just that—information. It's largely benign, often insignificant (insofar as it may not yet be understood and may not affect our life choices), and far more ambiguous than it used to be. It's also a great deal more complex than it seemed to be even just a few years ago. But we can turn complexity to our advantage. If we engage with our DNA and try to understand it, to leverage the nuances of genetic influence as opportunity rather than fate, we can incorporate genetic knowledge as a variable in our decision making, helping us to make early, informed, and open choices.

III.

THERE'S ANOTHER PROBLEM with treating genetic information as something toxic or dangerous to us. It turns out that, even when a test brings bad news, we might not actually be devastated. Consider Alzheimer's disease.

Alzheimer's is an especially terrifying neurological illness. It is marked by waves of dementia that increase in length and severity. People with Alzheimer's might, in the first few years of the disease, seem like their normal selves nearly all the time, but there are frightening interruptions of mental anguish. Gradually, the disease takes away the most important parts of our lives: our memories, our relationships, and our senses of who we are. Parents forget their children, spouses reject their mates. Making the experience even worse, a paranoia often swoops in during these spells, so Alzheimer's patients lash out in fear and contempt at those they may, in more settled periods, recognize and adore. Once the illness reveals symptoms, it typically takes years until the lucid times become the exception, each year being marked by a further decline. Death for an Alzheimer's patient may not come for several years after diagnosis, and it usually results from another condition, such as pneumonia. While there are some treatments that may slow the symptoms of the disease—the anxiety, the aggression—there's nothing that can stop it or reverse it. And there are no proven preventive measures.

As in many neurological conditions, DNA can play a large role in who develops Alzheimer's disease. Among other genetic associations, people with a variation in their *APOE* gene can have a significantly higher chance of developing the disease. This risk is not definitive—

people can have a risky *APOE* variation and not develop dementia. But it can be a very strong association, giving those who have it on a heterogeneous gene (meaning the variation occurs on just one side of the DNA helix) up to 5 times the average chance and those who have it on a homogeneous gene (when the variation occurs on both sides of the helix) up to 15 times the risk. This can increase one's lifetime chance of developing Alzheimer's to as much as a 70 percent certainty.

Because the risk swings so widely and isn't absolute, the line from the medical establishment has been to recommend *against* testing people for an *APOE* variation that predisposes them to developing Alzheimer's. Panel after panel has delivered this consensus opinion. "Neither predictive nor diagnostic genetic testing for susceptibility genes (e.g., *APOE*) should be encouraged," a panel of Stanford University and other Bay Area bioethicists recommended in a 1998 *Nature Medicine* paper, arguing that *some* chance of developing Alzheimer's was too little justification to open Pandora's box.

Many such panels argue, moreover, that because there's no known treatment for Alzheimer's, testing should be discouraged. The reasoning comes down to a rule of thumb in medicine known as *test to treat*, which holds that medicine should test for only those diseases it can treat. If there's no effective treatment or preventive, the thinking goes, then the knowledge isn't of any use and can only cause harm. These recommendations were, for the most part, established in the 1990s, when the first warnings about genetic information being toxic knowledge began to solidify into policy statements.

But surprisingly, this notion that DNA can be destructive had never been examined scientifically, despite being codified into a doctrine among many geneticists and physicians. Though it seemed grounded in good science, there was no evidence that genetic information is, in fact, dangerous. What's more, there was no information at all on how people react to a diagnosis of genetic risk, let alone any statistics on whether people want to know the information.

This ambiguity inspired the REVEAL (pithy shorthand for Risk Evaluation and Education for Alzheimer's Disease) study. The idea behind REVEAL is pretty much what its name promises: finding out what happens when the genetic risk for Alzheimer's is revealed. How do people react? What actions do they take? And do they wish they'd never found out?

The study is the brainchild of Robert Green, MD, a physician and Alzheimer's expert at Boston University. Dr. Green, who comes across as an exceedingly genial and curious fellow, is an odd duck in the world of medical genetics. Green came to the field of genetics in the late 1990s, when he was already well along in his career doing Alzheimer's research. So he harbored none of the dogmatic rules and sectarian strictures of bioethics when he started to wonder if people might find their *APOE* status informative. Thinking that the reasonable way to find out would be to ask them, he proposed a research study that would divulge *APOE* status and then assess whether people found knowing their risk to be helpful. But he was entirely unprepared for the reaction from bioethicists and geneticists. "Everyone just shrank back in horror," he says. "They thought it would be irresponsible and unethical to divulge that."

Dr. Green, a man of greater patience than many, persisted and spent several years navigating a formidable number of obstacles and objections in search of funding from the National Institutes of Health (NIH). "It's been notable how much crap I've gotten simply for asking the question and trying to find the answer in an ethical way," Dr. Green says with a smile.

In 1999, the NIH agreed to fund Dr. Green's study to answer the question: What do people do when they learn they have an increased genetic risk for a disease? Dr. Green and his fellow researchers contacted dozens of adults who had a parent with Alzheimer's, identifying 162 who were willing to be tested for an *APOE* variation. After drawing a bit of blood, the researchers tested the subjects' DNA. Patients were told two numbers: one indicating whether they were positive for an *APOE* variation, and the other quantifying their lifetime risk for developing the disease, a figure derived by combining the nature of their variation (heterozygous or homozygous) with a few personal factors (gender, race, family history). The results were delivered to the participants with great care: A genetic counselor walked each individual through every permutation of the data, and all the subjects had several follow-up appointments with counselors; therapists were also on call.

All this support was necessary because the genetics experts who'd vetted the study design had been convinced that significant numbers of people would be thrown, if not altogether devastated, by the results. "People were predicting catastrophic reactions from as many as 1 in 10 subjects," Dr. Green recalls. "Depression, suicide, quitting their jobs, abandoning their families. They were anticipating the worst."

But that isn't what happened at all. By nearly every measure, people told their risk for developing Alzheimer's disease later in life did not plunge into depression, give up hope, abandon their families, or lose their purpose in life. Instead, they seemed to process the information, integrate it into their lives, and take some actions directed at preventing the disease (since there are no proven preventives out there, this typically amounts to living generally healthier lives as well as taking nutritional supplements such as vitamin E, which some people believe may slow progression, though there's little evidence behind that). Intriguingly, these actions seemed to correlate strongly with the volume of risk. Specifically, Dr. Green's team found a 1 to 5 correlation between risk and behavior—for every 1 percent higher risk a person had for developing Alzheimer's, he or she was 5 percent more likely to make certain positive behavior changes.

All in all, Dr. Green says, these people seemed to adopt a greater dedication to enjoying and appreciating their lives. "People are handling it," Dr. Green says. "It doesn't seem to be producing any clinically apparent distress."

The conclusion directly contradicts the conventional wisdom about how people use genetic information. Though the "test to treat" dogma assumes that the only purpose genetic information can have is medical, Dr. Green found that, beyond treatment, there are many other ways in which people will act on their results. People might change their investments, their insurance coverage, their long-term-care arrangements, and so on. Dr. Green categorizes these under the rubric of "personal utility." Sometimes the results were striking: Dr. Green had previously found that people with an increased risk of Alzheimer's were nearly six times more likely than those without it to increase their long-term-care insurance coverage. This finding was particularly unsettling to the long-term-care industry, as Dr. Green discovered when he spoke to a group of long-term-care insurers. "They were freaked out that people would have information that they could use to make choices, and that the insurers wouldn't have access to that information," Dr. Green recalls. "They were worried it was going to put them out of business."

But aside from insurers' future profits, was there any danger to having the knowledge? Did some people find that it hurt them more than it helped them? Not really. The study measured people's stress and discomfort using what's called an Impact of Event Scale (IES), a simple questionnaire that quantifies how much people are disturbed by new information. An IES score is a widely used surrogate for stress; it measures whether people find information intrusively unsettling (how much it keeps them up at night) and how much they *avoid* thinking about it.

Out of a total IES score of 75, a person getting above 19 is considered to be highly stressed. And the *APOE*-positive patients? "We did not find significant psychiatric distress," Dr. Green says. Those who tested positive for an *APOE* variation registered an 8.5 IES score, on average, somewhat higher than those who tested negative for the genetic risk but a full 10 points below a level considered clinically dangerous. When the survey was repeated a year or more later, people with a positive *APOE* result were about even with those who tested negative. They seemed to have processed the information, faced up to their risks, and moved on with their lives. In other words, people weren't reacting as horribly as the medical establishment had been certain they would.

The research has continued with a second and a third group of individuals, and with these groups, Dr. Green is further challenging the conventional wisdom about the perils of genetics. In one significant shift, for instance, Dr. Green is questioning the need for the layers of genetic counselors and therapists. "We're looking at what happens if you don't do this elaborate thing. What if you do it like a lab test in your doctor's office? And the answer is [that patients] do fine. We're treating it more like cholesterol and less like Huntington's disease."

The REVEAL study tells us more than just how people react to genetic information. It tells us something about how social norms happen.

We can't predict how people will react to information. And we can't mandate an appropriate level of concern from on high. The National Human Genome Research Institute began funding the Human Genome Project in the 1980s, and in the early 1990s, Francis Collins, MD, PhD, head of the organization from 1993 through 2008, set aside 5 percent of the project's $3 billion budget for exploring what's known as ELSI—ethical, legal, and social issues. Most of that went to the so-called experts known as bioethicists. One hundred and fifty million dollars is a lot to spend on philosophy, and it's no great surprise that no clear conclusions were made about what the ethics concerning genetic information should be.

Social norms don't develop according to what bioethicists decide is right or wrong. They aren't created by scientific committees and then delivered on parchment to be read at the Forum. Ethics happen because the opinion of society, in some collective process involving gut instincts and trade-offs, seems to coalesce around some basic principles. Dr. Green's REVEAL study (which actually got some of that ELSI money) showed that no matter what the experts may think will emerge as an ethical problem, real people may approach the issue in an entirely different way.

This is especially important because as the cost of testing drops and the usefulness of genetic knowledge increases, whole genome sequencing—taking a gander at all 6 billion bits of our DNA—will become a routine part of all medical treatment, just as genetic tests today are a routine part of pregnancy. It may start with our children or our grandchildren, but soon enough, everybody will get their entire genomes sequenced at birth. And then they'll be sequenced again at regular intervals, to see if any new mutations have raised our odds for cancer or other diseases. The issue won't be whether to look; it will be what to do with what's found. Everyone, in other words, will be facing decisions like Teri Smieja's; some of them will be direr, and many more will be more mundane. But they'll all require that we confront the idea of risk.

If society really wants to make the most of our science, truly wants to step toward preventive medicine and leverage all of our knowledge to its best effect, then genetics is a good place to start. It is, as science would say, the baseline—the ground floor from where we all begin our lives. But genetics isn't fate. What's coded in our DNA does not, most of the time, determine who we are or what will befall us. It plays a role but doesn't run the show. Most genetic influence isn't as dramatic as an *APOE* variation or a *BRCA* mutation. It's smaller stuff.

If we begin our Decision Trees with our genetics, with a consideration of what we're starting with, it can help us make better choices later. Genetics is powerful stuff. It can reveal all sorts of unexpected things. But it is the first clue we have to our health. Sixty years after the discovery of DNA, it's high time that the science be liberated and made relevant to all of us. That's the argument Dr. Watson, the codiscoverer of DNA, offered to a group of fellow geneticists at a conference in 2008. "I think we should use common sense, and get common information which can help the most people," he said. "Our aim should be to help the damned, and we should somehow un-damn them."

It's important to remember that Teri's quandary wasn't based on having breast cancer. Instead, it was based on her high *risk* of developing breast cancer, and her reactions to that risk could potentially improve and extend her life. What she wanted, really, was a way to factor her own circumstances—her age, her family circumstances and history, her options—into the body of science out there that set out the large, population-size implications. What she needed (and what we all will need) is a way to navigate through her decision. She described it like this: "It's all very complicated, and I'm learning a lot. I'm breaking it all down as it applies to me. I feel that I got a look at this scientific crystal ball. I kind of know my future, and now I can fix it."

DNA + Environment = You

Why Genetics Is Just the First Step
in Making Better Health Decisions

I.

IN THE SPRING OF 2005, Eddy Curry was a promising young basketball player for the Chicago Bulls. Drafted into the NBA at age 18,
Curry had struggled during his first couple of years in the league, just as
any teenager might. But standing 6 feet 11 inches tall, Curry was starting to come into his own in his third season—he was averaging a decent
16 points per game and grabbing his share of rebounds. He was the sort
of player teams build championships around.

So there was more than just Curry's health at stake one evening in
North Carolina when, warming up on the court before a game against
the Charlotte Hornets, he felt his heart racing much faster than normal.
Curry was whisked into the visitors' locker room and hooked up to a
heart monitor and then dispatched to the local hospital. The verdict:
Curry had had a bout of arrhythmia, an abnormal heartbeat that can
lead to a heart attack or stroke.

Curry's diagnosis immediately called to mind the tragic stories of
Hank Gathers and Reggie Lewis, two outstanding ballplayers who, in
1990 and 1993, respectively, collapsed on basketball courts and died. In
both cases, the cause was cardiac arrest brought on by hypertrophic

cardiomyopathy, or HCM, a condition in which the walls of the heart muscle have thickened, impeding bloodflow. HCM greatly increases the risk of sudden cardiac arrest, particularly during strenuous exertion, such as playing professional basketball. The condition occurs frequently in young people and is believed to be nearly always inherited—that is, a result of genetics. The fear was that Curry had HCM, too.

Curry was ordered to stop playing for 6 weeks and rest, effectively ending his season. He spent much of that time scurrying to various hospitals and cardiologists in Boston, Minneapolis, and Chicago for a dizzying sequence of tests and evaluations. The examinations revealed that Curry had an enlarged heart, but the evidence of HCM was inconclusive. In fact, several prominent cardiologists said his heart was sound and he was fit to play. Curry was eager to get back to his job and play basketball. "I'm cool now. The doctors said it's nothing life-threatening," Curry told reporters not long after the incident in Charlotte. But the Bulls weren't so sure; there was one more test they thought Curry should take: a genetic test for HCM.

HCM is most commonly caused by a mutation on one of a handful of genes. Though the precise mutation can differ from person to person, the result is the same: The gene overproduces muscle proteins, thickening the chamber walls of the heart muscle. Though HCM can be detected by an echocardiogram or other tests, the genetic *risk* for developing HCM can be established only with a DNA test. A positive test means that an individual has inherited the mutated gene and is almost assured of developing HCM—something on the order of 90 percent do—though the timing and severity can't be known.

When the next NBA season came around in September 2005, the Bulls offered Curry a new $5 million contract, with one condition attached: He had to test his DNA. If he didn't have the genetic mutation, he could take the contract and play with the team. (If he took the test and turned up positive, the Bulls promised to pay Curry $500,000 for 50 years.)

Though the team may have wanted Curry to think he had no choice in the matter, his Decision Tree actually looked a little different than the Bulls' ultimatum suggested. The team had actually presented him with a choice. He could take the test and perhaps stay with the Bulls. Or he could decide not to take the test and see if another NBA team might be willing to sign him up. If he did take the test and it turned up positive, there was yet a larger choice facing Curry: He could look for another team, continue to play basketball, and risk dying on the court. Or he could drop the sport, avoid strenuous activity in general, and increase his chances of living a long and uneventful life. With the new basketball season looming, Curry had a lot to consider.

II.

TO BETTER UNDERSTAND THE ROLE that genetics will play in our health care, I visited Harvard Medical School in Boston on a bright morning in the summer of 2007 and sat in on a peculiar meeting. On the third floor of the New Research Building—a hulking glass structure that looks like its architects turned it inside out—George Church, PhD, the director of Harvard's Center for Computational Genetics, had gathered a select group of 10 academics, physicians, and entrepreneurs. These 10 were the first of a legion of individuals who will willingly give up their DNA, along with their complete medical histories, in order to learn something about themselves—and help push medicine into the future. These were the first members of the Personal Genome Project, or PGP, Dr. Church's effort to create a library of 100,000 human genomes and shake out some of the complexity that lies in our genetic codes.

It was just past 8:00 a.m., and as the 10 lingered over coffee and pastries, waiting for the meeting to officially start, a lab technician entered the room and took them, one by one, into a nearby office to draw samples of their blood. The samples were sent to a lab, where the DNA would later be extracted and analyzed. That DNA would help them write the story of how they became who they are—and what they may need to heed in the future.

Soon enough, Dr. Church arrived and called the meeting to order. A tall man of 6 feet 4 inches, with a booming voice and a bushy, pioneer-style beard, Dr. Church can seem imposing from afar. But talk to him and he comes across as soft-spoken and patient, admirable qualities for

Eddy Curry's Decision Tree

When NBA star Eddy Curry was diagnosed with arrhythmia and an enlarged heart, there was concern he was at risk for the genetic condition known as hypertrophic cardiomyopathy, or HCM. There was one way to find out: He could take a DNA test for the condition. Only problem was, if he tested positive, his career may have been over. Here's his hypothetical Decision Tree.

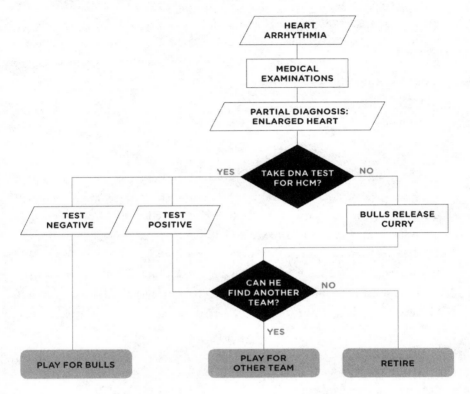

somebody who's at least 6 months ahead of the rest of the world when it comes to genetics.

Dr. Church explains the PGP like this: Our DNA is a map for who we are and what we will become. But DNA is just the blueprint; it's only the starting point. The environment also plays a significant role in our development and our health, from what our mothers eat when we're in the womb to whether we're exposed to asbestos in our thirties. Dr. Church, being a scientist, prefers to express it with an equation that looks like this:

$$DNA + Environment = You$$

The idea is that the more we understand about how our genomes interplay with our environments—our diets, our exercise, the amount of sleep we get, the chemicals we're exposed to—the better we'll be able to understand and influence our health. And the PGP is an effort to create a model, using data from 100,000 volunteers, for how that can be done. "People assume that medicine is all deterministic, that it's set in stone. But it's not," Dr. Church tells me later. "Most of medicine is probabilistic. It's an estimate of likelihoods, based on our best available research. Genetics can help improve those probabilities. It can give us better odds."

In contrast to genetic testing, which looks at small regions of single genes for specific disease variations, the PGP plans to sequence the entire genomes of its members—all 6 billion base pairs of DNA for each individual. In the 1990s, it took just under $3 billion to sequence the single whole genome in the Human Genome Project, but Dr. Church's lab has developed technology that can do whole-genome sequencing for a fraction of that. It's a daunting goal, one that would dramatically change the landscape of genetics if it's accomplished.

But genetics is just half of what the PGP is after. If the "DNA" part of Dr. Church's equation is your genome, the "You" part is what's known as your phenome, a term that encompasses everything about your physical body. Whereas your genotype is defined as a characteristic of your

DNA, your phenotype is a physical characteristic, the end result of the interplay between genes and environment. And while measuring the genome can be done with some blood and a machine, measuring phenomes takes a bit more work. It means asking a lot of questions and taking a lot of notes. For instance, all of us know our heights, weights, and eye colors. Fewer of us know our arm spans or resting blood pressures. But who among us knows the directions of our hair whorls or the Gell-Coombs types of our allergies? The PGP tallies head circumferences, injuries, chin clefts and cheek dimples, whether volunteers can roll their tongues or hyperflex their joints, whether they dislike hot climates or are hot tempered, if they've often been exposed to power lines or wood dust or diesel exhaust or textile fibers. The PGP questionnaire asks how many meals participants eat a day and whether they prefer their food fried, broiled, or barbecued. It even demands an accounting of how much television they watch. And, perhaps most important, PGP volunteers hand over most aspects of their medical histories, from vaccines to prescriptions.

The reason for the interrogation is simple: The longer the questionnaire—meaning the more phenotypic information the PGP can gather—the more powerful Dr. Church's equation becomes. One hundred thousand sounds like a lot of people. But say you're looking at Parkinson's disease: Maybe only 1,000 of those 100,000 have it, and of those 1,000 only 100 or 40 or 30 may have a particular genetic variation that may (or may not) have some influence on the disease. Suddenly, a massive study has become a rather small data set. One hundred thousand isn't so many people after all.

This massive amount of data is a good thing. Part of the genius of the PGP is that it's not just one research study, not just one experiment, but a database that can be crunched and recrunched again and again. The PGP, in effect, automates the research process. Scientists can simply choose a category of phenotype and a possible genetic correlation, and statistically significant associations should flow out of the data like honey from a hive. A genetic predisposition for colon cancer, for instance, might be found to lead to disease in conjunction with a diet high in barbecued foods, or a certain form of heart disease might be associated with a particular gene and exposure to a particular virus. Genomic discovery isn't a research problem anymore. It's a search function.

There's one other significant difference between the PGP and most traditional genetics research: openness. PGP volunteers are not just subjects, they're also participants. Once the database gets large enough—once the pool of volunteers expands from 10 to 1,000 to 10,000 and on toward 100,000—the information won't just inform scientists about population traits and characteristics. It will also tell the PGP participants things about their own histories and futures. In an admirable gesture of openness, any results that spool out of a participant's information will be returned to them. So, for instance, if a researcher uses a volunteer's information to establish a link between some genetic sequence and a risk of disease, the volunteer will have that information communicated to him. This, alas, is not at all the norm for genetic research, in which the standard practice is to *never* return information to a study's participants and to "de-identify" every scrap of data so it can't be linked back to one individual, no matter what.

For PGP volunteers, this openness means they must sign on to a principle Dr. Church calls open consent, which goes a step further than the standard informed consent whereby study subjects acknowledge that they know what they're getting into. Open consent acknowledges that, even when subjects' names will be removed to make the data anonymous, there's no promise of absolute confidentiality. As Dr. Church sees it, any guarantee of privacy is false; there is no way to ensure that a malevolent soul won't tap into a system and, once there, manage to extract bits of personal information. After all, even de-identified data are subject to misuse: Latanya Sweeney, PhD, a computer scientist at Carnegie Mellon University in Pittsburgh, demonstrated the ease of "re-identification" by cross-referencing "anonymized" health insurance records with voter registration rolls. (She found former Massachusetts governor William Weld's medical files by searching for his birth date, zip code, and sex.)

Such openness may seem like a radical gesture in an age of privacy fears, especially fears about our health histories. But to Dr. Church, open consent isn't just a philosophy, it's also practical. If the PGP were locked down by privacy restrictions, it would be far less valuable as a data source for research, and the pace of research using it would accordingly be much slower. By making the information open and available, Dr. Church hopes to draw curious scientists to the data to pursue their own questions and reach their own insights. The potential fields of inquiry range from medicine to genealogy, forensics, and general biology. "The ground is changing right underneath them," he says of the medical establishment. "Right now, there's a wall between clinical research and clinical practice. The science isn't jumping over. The PGP is what clinical practice would be like if the research actually made it to the patient."

Even among PGP participants, this level of science and openness can be rather intimidating. That's why Dr. Church insisted that the first 10 volunteers for the PGP all have backgrounds in medicine or genetics. It's a smart group that includes John Halamka, MD, the chief information officer of Harvard Medical School and a physician; Rosalynn Gill, PhD, the chief science officer at Sciona (a company that gives personalized health and nutrition advice based on one's genetics); Steven Pinker, PhD, a noted psychologist and author; Esther Dyson, a technology investor (in 23andMe, among other companies) and personalized health care evangelist; and Dr. Church himself. (Such credentials aren't required of the other 99,990 participants, though they do have to pass a difficult genetics literacy quiz to demonstrate informed consent.)

That summer morning in Boston, the conversation was tinged with anxiety. What would happen, participants wanted to know, with their samples? If somebody were hell-bent on misusing their DNA, planting it at a crime scene, say, could they? And how long would it be until they got some personally relevant information out of their participation? The PGP 10 batted these questions around for most of the day. Dr. Church mostly listened, but occasionally reassured the group, in his calm baritone, that no, no outside researchers would have access to the blood samples and that yes, while it might be technically possible for somebody to reconstruct their DNA, few labs on earth were capable of such a thing. And about whether the data would have any individual utility at all, Dr. Church offered his own example. After he posted his own medical history on his Web site a couple of years ago, someone who happened to look at it suggested that he ask his doctor about his heart medication—the dose looked wrong. Sure enough, it was, and Dr. Church changed his dose. "You all know what you're getting into," Dr. Church told the group that day. "We're all going to die of something, and the closer we get to that, by way of genetics, the more we know about our destiny."

As the day progressed, the conversation turned away from the logistics of the project and toward the fun stuff: what they'd do once they got a peek at their genomes. Some wondered how they'd have to change their diets and habits, others fretted over telling their families about various disease risks, and none were sure that their doctors would have a clue about what to do with the information. As I sat there listening to them reckon with the future they'd signed on for, I had my own realization. Though the group wasn't likely to be mistaken for the Mercury Seven (plus three), in their tweedy way they had something in common with the astronauts who 50 years earlier had manned the first US space program. These 10 were genetic explorers, catapulting themselves into the future.

By doing the hard math that will tease out how DNA and the environment interact, the PGP will be something we can all learn from, whether or not we sign on ourselves. The science that comes out of the project will illuminate how specific genetic variations can play out along several different decision pathways, depending on the choices and behaviors of individuals. These patterns might guide our own decisions, helping us think about how we want to live our lives, what sacrifices today are worth what results tomorrow. The PGP will make it easier for each of us to understand his or her own Decision Trees.

Given enough time and participants, the PGP could even help somebody like Eddy Curry. If statistics hold, there will be hundreds of people in the study with arrhythmia. And since HCM occurs in about 1 out of every 500 people, the PGP may wind up with as many as 200 individuals with a genetic risk of that condition. That's enough people to reveal patterns between genetic risk, behaviors, and overall health. In other words, if some number of people with an HCM risk choose to stay active and play sports, we might see how many eventually suffer a cardiac event.

And of those with an HCM risk who opt to avoid strenuous activity, we might see how many are still struck by heart attacks. With enough data and a few calculations, the PGP could provide answers relevant to Curry's and an infinite number of other decisions.

In late 2008, the PGP 10 got the first glimpse of their information. Among the 10 volunteers, some had an increased risk for prostate cancer, some had possible risks for neurological conditions, one even had a strong chance of something called Charcot-Marie-Tooth disease. And one member of the PGP 10, it seems, has a genetic mutation that predisposes him for HCM.

III.

READING YOUR GENOMIC PROFILE—learning your predispositions for various diseases, odd traits, and a talent or two—is something like going to a phantasmagorical family reunion. First, you're introduced to the grandfather who died of an early cancer decades before you were born. Then you move along for a chat with your parents, who are uncharacteristically happy to talk about their health—Dad's prostate, Mom's digestive tract. Next, you have the odd experience of getting acquainted with future versions of yourself from 10 or 20 or 30 years down the road. Finally, you face the prospect of telling your children that they probably face an increased genetic risk for whatever you inherited from your parents.

The experience is simultaneously unsettling, illuminating, and empowering. And it's one that more people are having every day. Since 2007, a new industry allows anyone with the curiosity and a few hundred dollars to get a peek at their genomes, and to do it without a doctor's prescription or permission. This is the age of personal genomics, represented most prominently by two Silicon Valley companies, Navigenics and 23andMe. In contrast to traditional genetic testing, a closed system dominated by giant diagnostic companies that require physician approval and operate under strict government regulatory oversight, the personal genomics business is selling its services straight to consumers.

And befitting its Silicon Valley roots, the industry has turned genetics into a people-friendly technology with all the answers of Google and the networking potential of Facebook.

The founding principle of personal genomics is to give people access to a deeper understanding of who they are, to provide information that can inform or improve the way they live. "If I tell you you've got a genetic likelihood of getting colon cancer, you're going to get a colonoscopy early," says David Agus, MD, a prominent Los Angeles oncologist and the cofounder of Navigenics. "And that's going to save lives."

But personal genomics has proven to be a lightning-rod industry, one that makes health regulators, doctors, and even many geneticists nervous. The science is too new, critics argue, the information too sketchy, the ambiguity too great, and the oversight too slight. Ordinary individuals, the argument goes, won't know what to do with their DNA information. Better to wait, they say, until the scientists have figured out what it all means and physicians can help them make sense of it.

But like it or not, genetics is no longer a field that can be contained by the scientists or the doctors. Navigenics and 23andMe have liberated genetic information for the masses (or at least those masses who can afford their services), and they have created a profound choice: Now any ordinary person can opt to look at her genome, get some inkling of how her DNA may influence her health, and take a step toward the future of medicine. Or she can choose not to and stay within the comfortable confines of conventional medicine. Either way, the choice is ours, not a doctor's or the government's or an employer's. And while that choice seems novel today, tomorrow it will be entirely ordinary. In a few years, or perhaps in a decade or so, genetics will be part of every thorough health assessment, offering a baseline understanding of what we're made of. It will be as familiar a data point as cholesterol and blood pressure levels are today.

It works like this: Log on to 23andMe's Web site, fill in your credit card information, and register for a genetic scan. A few days later, a test tube will arrive at your door. Spend about 10 minutes spitting into it—it takes a surprising amount of spit to fill the tube—and send it back. A couple of weeks later, you'll get an e-mail: Your results are ready. A few clicks later, you'll have insight into how your genes influence your risk for developing dozens of conditions and diseases, from diabetes to heart disease to restless legs syndrome. No doctor or prescription required.

23andMe charges $499, which buys you identification of about 550,000 SNPs, those one-letter code sequences of ACTG in our DNA (see Chapter 2). Navigenics charges $999 for its test and uses a similar SNP-based approach.

23andMe opened for business in November 2007, and the timing was impeccable. Eric Lander, PhD, the founding director of the Broad Institute of MIT and Harvard and one of the principal architects of the Human Genome Project, called 2007 the "annus mirabilis" of genetics research. The cause was the explosion of genome-wide association studies, or GWAS, a new kind of study design that compares a group of people who have a disease with an SNP scan of multiple genomes, looking for possible common associations between the disease and the DNA.

The GWAS fall somewhere between traditional genetic research, which concentrates on specific portions of DNA, and the blunderbuss approach of the PGP, which will compare entire genomes against huge breakdowns of physical traits. The GWAS take a middle road by starting with a disease with an imprecise genetic component—type 2 diabetes or Crohn's disease, for example—and looking at several hundred thousand SNPs scattered across the genome, hoping to identify common patterns.

The hypothesis behind most GWAS research is that certain variations from one person to another—a C in me, say, where most people have a T—can have significant implications for human health. The torrent of GWAS in 2007, then, was the first effort to associate the most common diseases of our age with possible genetic influences. "Suddenly we have the tools to apply to any problem: cancer, diabetes—a huge list of diseases," Dr. Lander told me enthusiastically. "It's just a stunning explosion of data. Pick a metaphor: We've now landed on this new continent and the people are out there exploring it, and we're finding mountains and waterfalls and rivers. We're turning on lights in dark rooms. We're finding pieces to the jigsaw puzzle."

Even the sober *New England Journal of Medicine* described trying to keep up with the research as "drinking from the fire hose." The catch, though, is that GWAS are not designed to inform clinical practice in the doctor's office; they are designed to suss out genetic links at a population level, not an individual level. They're a good way to learn about a disease in general, but they haven't been proven to have specific implications for individuals. And that's the leap that 23andMe and Navigenics are making: By taking the research directly to me and you, they're leapfrogging over the normal (some would say plodding) pace of scientific advancement with a promising but imperfect technology (an SNP analysis, for instance, doesn't reveal a risk for HCM, though the 23andMe results do reveal a genetic variation that's been associated with improved athletic performance).

Which raises the question: If scientists and physicians are having trouble keeping up with genetic research, how are you and I supposed to make sense of the information? After all, joining a personal genomics service isn't like joining Facebook. There's nothing intuitive about navigating your genome; it requires not just a new vocabulary but also a new conception of personhood. Scrape below the skin and we're flesh and bone; scrape below that and we're code.

Both 23andMe and Navigenics have teams of geneticists on staff to filter through the confusing world of research papers and studies and identify what they regard as valid research that's worthy of their customers' attention. 23andMe's Web site, for instance, interprets more than 100 conditions and their genetic components, while Navigenics runs down the genetic risks for about 28 conditions, as of this writing. Each company, in turn, automatically matches this information to each customer's results, offering a customized interpretation of what the research implies. In other words, each customer is able to navigate the vast body of scientific research on a tailor-made tour, using his or her own genome as a map. The experience is slick and polished; it's hard to imagine how one could make genetic science any friendlier. The hope is that the experience eliminates false alarms and lets customers trust the science. Maybe even enjoy it.

THE ARRIVAL OF PERSONAL GENOMICS took the traditional medical establishment—regulators, insurers, doctors—by surprise. Prior to their launches, both 23andMe and Navigenics had approached the Food and Drug Administration, which regulates diagnostic genetic testing, regarding their business strategies. But the agency offered no explicit guidance for navigating the gray area between information and diagnosis. That left regulation up to the states—and some have shown more concern than others.

Within 6 months of 23andMe having opened for business, public health departments in both New York and California reacted negatively to personal genomics. State officials sent cease-and-desist letters to the companies, warning them that they were in violation of regulations governing diagnostic testing. The states were particularly concerned that the tests were being conducted without a physician's order. California regulators went a step further, warning that giving people access to so much information without a physician intermediary was unnecessarily creating a group of people one regulator characterized as the "worried well. Once they get the results, they don't know what to do about it."

But information that is coupled *with* some guidance on what to do with it can be a boon to our health; it can improve our decisions. And while guidance was once available only from a physician, the great opportunity offered by personal genomics and many other tools discussed in this book is our new ability to secure guidance from many sources. 23andMe and Navigenics both meet this standard of reputability; they take their science and their obligation to their customers seriously and treat the subjects carefully. There are, of course, many other companies selling genetic tests directly to consumers. Even Amway has gotten into the game, offering genetic tests from a company called Interleukin Genetics that purport to tell people how well they metabolize B vitamins and whether they're at risk for heart inflammation. The tests, which cost between $100 and $200, are described in exactly the sort of deterministic language that Dr. Church and public health departments are wary of.

Within a few months of issuing its cease-and-desist letters, the

California Department of Public Health had reached an understanding with 23andMe and Navigenics that allowed the companies to offer tests directly to Californians. New York State still requires a physician intermediary, so 23andMe no longer offers the test to New Yorkers. Navigenics has arranged to work through physicians in the state.

But physicians, it turns out, have been just as unprepared for personal genomics as the government—and often just as defensive about it. The *New England Journal of Medicine* has called the services premature and suggested that doctors tell curious patients to "ask again in a few years" until the medical profession has figured out the science. Meanwhile, the American Medical Association, the largest group of doctors in the United States, in 2008 issued a statement critical of direct-to-consumer genetic testers like 23andMe, stating that "the potential for patients to be harmed by [direct-to-consumer] genetic tests is magnified without a physician acting as a learned intermediary" and recommending that "clinical testing should be performed under the care of a qualified health care professional."

There's something disingenuous about both of these arguments. The notion that medical science will, at some point in the future, settle out once and for all what genetics can tell us and it should only then be revealed to individuals is at best wishful thinking. By its very nature, medicine is an inexact science, one that never operates with absolute certainty. As Dr. Church says, it is a probabilistic, rather than deterministic, discipline. In that regard, personal genomics, with its typically modest percentages of increased or decreased risk for disease, is just like any other risk factor for disease—a statistical estimate rather than a certainty.

And the argument that doctors are expert gatekeepers to genetic information is likewise a fabulist invention. The medical establishment has been woefully slow and recalcitrant about integrating genetics into clinical practice. Though most med students get some instruction in genetics, few doctors in the United States go so far as board certification in genetics: They number just more than 1,000, according to the American Board of Medical Genetics. Indeed, genetic education among doctors has increased because of personal genomics; Navigenics even sponsors continuing-education programs on the topic for physicians. In this sense, 23andMe and Navigenics are doing consumers and medicine a service by pushing genetics into the examination room, compelling doctors to get up to speed on the personal implications of genetics research.

Geneticists, meanwhile, have raised their own red flags about personal genomics, arguing that direct-to-consumer services go too far in implying that the research is ready for individuals to use. David Goldstein, PhD, the director of the Center for Human Genome Variation at Duke University's Institute for Genome Sciences and Policy, has been perhaps the most prominent critic in this regard; his argument boils down to a critique of the limitations of SNP analysis. While the torrent of GWAS has produced lots of tantalizing hints at genetic associations, he says, they have done a poor job of drawing out real associations between our genomes and diseases, making them flimsy grounding for individual action. The effects found so far are so slight as to be useless for informing individual health—and all the ones yet to be found, he suggests, are likely even weaker. "Even though genomewide association studies have worked better and faster than expected," he wrote in a commentary in the *New England Journal of Medicine,* "they have not explained as much of the genetic component of many diseases and conditions as was anticipated."

But Dr. Goldstein's critique shouldn't be mistaken for an indictment of the *idea* of personal genomics. Indeed, the fact that the science is a moving target and the technology is steadily improving should be an argument that compels people toward understanding what DNA is and how it influences our health—and doing so sooner rather than later. Because whether you decide to learn about your genome now or put it off for a few years, sooner or later we'll all be making decisions based on our DNA.

SO YOU'VE GOT YOUR GENOME. Now what?

To answer that question, let me give you a rundown of what 23andMe told me about my health and what I did with it.

23andMe's analysis told me that I have a genetic variation that increases my risk for exfoliation glaucoma, raising it to about seven times the average American's risk. That puts my lifetime risk of the disease somewhere around 15 percent—a not-impossible fate. With that information in hand, I visited my eye doctor and told him about the fate. At first, he was a bit taken aback; I was the first patient he'd seen who came bearing a printout warning of a genetic risk for an eye disease. But as he took a look at the sheet that 23andMe provides that discusses the risk and the disease, he nodded, smiled, and proceeded with my eye exam. After I read the eye chart and followed the path of his light pen, he performed the test for glaucoma by checking the pressure inside my eyeballs. It was, he said, a routine test he surely would've done in any case. It seemed normal. "There's nothing else I can suggest," he told me, "except to be sure to make regular appointments."

23andMe also told me I have higher risks of obesity and type 2 diabetes than average. There's not much danger there, since I play the environmental side of Dr. Church's DNA + Environment equation pretty thoroughly already: I exercise several times a week and maintain a lean weight. But again, those are signals that I shouldn't let up as I get older.

My results revealed one more tidbit to file away for the future: I have a genetic variation that appears to substantially increase my risk of having muscle pain known as myopathy while taking certain statin drugs. Since my bad cholesterol is low and my good cholesterol is blessedly high, that's not an issue today. But in a few years, if my cholesterol creeps up—as it does for most people—and my doctor recommends a statin drug, that information may help me select the right kind.

Those are some of the downsides. 23andMe also suggests some potential upsides in my DNA. My genes may offer me some protection against colorectal cancer (that made me think, perhaps counterproductively, that maybe I don't have to cut back on red meat) and gout (ditto with ice cream). My scan also tells me that I have reduced risks of celiac disease and Crohn's disease, which is welcome news.

All told, the influences are small, amounting to a few percentage points' higher risk here or a couple ticks' lower risk there. The information is intriguing but not altogether life changing, which is pretty much what Dr. Church and others said would be the case.

For someone looking to his genome to inform his actions, the best answer may be to go ahead and look, but don't do anything rash. In nearly all cases, there's no reason to do anything at all. Genetics rarely contains information that demands immediate action; after all, you've been living with this stuff since birth anyway.

This point was made to me by Meredith Goldsmith, a decision analyst at Google. Goldsmith has a Stanford PhD in operations research, an obscure quantitative discipline that roughly involves analyzing complex systems and identifying strategic options; suffice it to say that it combines a lot of computer power and a lot of brainpower with the goal of making the best possible decisions. Several years ago, Dr. Goldsmith worked at a hedge fund where she designed computer models to identify when the firm should buy or sell various equities. One of the most overlooked considerations in finance, she realized, was the value of time—and specifically, of delay. "It wasn't just how much can I make if I buy today. Sometimes the smarter thing to do was to look at how much you could make by waiting to buy tomorrow. The point is, most decisions aren't one-time-only, now-or-never decisions." The value of waiting, Dr. Goldsmith says, is that in the future, more and better information may be available—information that actually improves your odds of making a good decision.

A similar idea applies, Dr. Goldsmith says, in making medical decisions, particularly those based on our genetics. "In finance, the value of delay is that you might get a better price in the future by waiting for some of the demand or supply to reappear. But in medical care it is the value of information that makes delay sometimes a better option."

It comes down to a bet on better numbers: The risk factors and predictions of future risk that a genetic scan may produce may, in time, turn into much different figures. Given a few years' delay, life and science may change enough that a decision that looks plain today may look much different tomorrow. "People may take a course of action that's irreversible like surgery, or unproven like an experimental drug. What seems to be missing is the probability that there will be more information later. But in 5 or 10 years, there could be new information that changes the way you might consider a decision." Dr. Goldsmith argues that genetic data is too often perceived as creating *one* opportunity for action—when the information is first received. But genetics actually creates a series of opportunities for action. "Given a known cost now—surgery—versus an uncertain cost in future—maybe a better treatment or a cure—we should consider the possibility that maybe that cost won't be necessary at all."

EDDY CURRY DIDN'T HAVE THE LUXURY OF WAITING. He had to decide. And sometime near the beginning of October 2005, he had. He didn't want to know.

Curry rejected the Chicago Bulls' ultimatum and decided not to take the genetic test for HCM. Curry opted to put himself on the open market, hopeful that some other team might offer him a contract. They were free to scrutinize his abilities, his stats, even his medical records, but they couldn't look at his genome. "It was a touchy situation," Curry said later. "I didn't think that my career should have rested on a DNA test."

As it turned out, another team was willing to take a chance on Curry and his heart. In early October 2005, he was traded to the New York Knicks. At first, Curry did well in New York, scoring an average of nearly 20 points a game in the 2006–2007 season. But within a couple of years, health problems again began to dog the ballplayer. Only this time, it wasn't his heart, it was his weight. At 350 pounds, Curry was too heavy for his frame, and he began to suffer knee injuries. He played only three games in the 2008–2009 season and was dispatched to a weight-loss clinic for the summer.

In other words, DNA no doubt played a large part in getting Curry to the NBA. But it's been less of a factor in recent years than his environment—in particular, how much he was eating. Though the outcome may not serve him well, Curry was right and the Bulls were wrong: He didn't need to look at his DNA. But he should've paid more attention to things he could control, starting with his diet.

It goes back to Dr. Church's equation: DNA + Environment = You. For most Americans, this calculation happens without our even knowing about it. It results in fairly good health and a life span stretching into our seventies. For most of the past century, medicine has been focused on the environment part of the equation—the stuff we could see and sometimes

How Genetics Influences Risks for Disease

A DNA scan by 23andMe allows for a personalized evaluation of risk for disease—though the actual effects are still rather small. Here are the author's risks for some conditions.

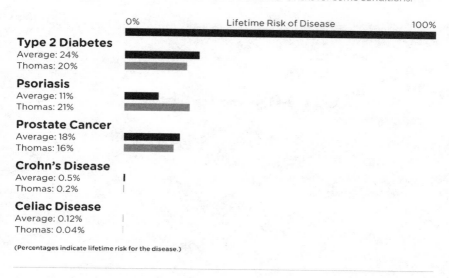

| | 0% | Lifetime Risk of Disease | 100% |

Type 2 Diabetes
Average: 24%
Thomas: 20%

Psoriasis
Average: 11%
Thomas: 21%

Prostate Cancer
Average: 18%
Thomas: 16%

Crohn's Disease
Average: 0.5%
Thomas: 0.2%

Celiac Disease
Average: 0.12%
Thomas: 0.04%

(Percentages indicate lifetime risk for the disease.)

influence. There's no doubt that adding DNA to the formula makes it a more complicated calculus. But it also becomes a more powerful one, because there are more factors that we can consider and address.

In my case, knowing my genome may not lead to any life-altering decisions. For most people, it probably shouldn't anyway. But by making our health a more explicit calculation, a genetic scan can be an important first step in a well-considered Decision Tree. Whatever it is that gets us thinking about our health early, *before* we succumb to symptoms and *before* we're locked into years of poor health habits—whether it's genetics, a false symptom, or a friend's diagnosis, it doesn't much matter. Thinking about what lies before us and what we can do to have better health—in other words, starting to think in terms of a Decision Tree— may be the most significant decision of all.

4

Change Is Hard

Why Behavior Change Is the Best Health Decision We Can Make, and Why It's the Hardest One, Too

I.

IN THE LATE 1950S, New York City's Department of Health offered to put its citizens on a diet. With a strong link emerging between obesity and heart disease, Norman Jolliffe, MD, of the department's bureau of nutrition, created what he called the Prudent Diet—a low-fat, reduced-calorie program that had shown promise in lowering weight. As diets went, it was decidedly not glamorous or gimmicky. There was a prosaic emphasis on calorie restriction: By taking in 200 to 300 calories fewer than one's metabolism required in a day, the typical individual might lose a pound a week. This meant there were no quick results, but it created a slow and steady process of loss that, Dr. Jolliffe believed, was the key to lasting weight loss and better health. The wisdom of the approach was borne out in a subsequent study, and in 1961, the city set up obesity clinics around the five boroughs that introduced citizens to the principles of the Prudent Diet. One of those clinics was in Kips Bay, a neighborhood in midtown Manhattan. Among the people who signed up there was a housewife from Queens named Jean Nidetch.

Then 38 years old, Nidetch was a woman of small stature but wide girth, weighing more than 200 pounds. She was, in almost every way, a typical overweight woman: She wanted to lose weight, she knew she should lose weight, but she just couldn't find a program she could stick with. Indeed, she lost weight all the time. "I became a professional dieter," she said later, keeping a collection of various diets in scrapbooks and old shoeboxes. At first, the Prudent Diet seemed to work for Nidetch, and she shed a few pounds. But the program was unforgiving and unfriendly, and, once again, she felt her will waning. She feared that she was going to lapse into obesity again. She needed help.

One afternoon, Nidetch invited some friends to her house. These women were also trying to lose a pound or 2 or 20. Nidetch told them about the program, that it seemed worthwhile but was tough. Together, she proposed, they might follow the rules of the Prudent Diet but adapt them to suit their lives. Along the way, they'd offer each other support and encouragement and help each other keep on track. "I thought if I could get my friends to go along with me, to stick to the diet too, maybe we'd all be able to make it together."

After just a few meetings, her small group had turned into several groups of women as word spread about this nifty group that was actually helping its members lose weight. Nidetch realized she was onto something special. The meetings she'd convened were more than a group—they fostered a philosophy that could get people to stick with a diet in a way they might not on their own. Soon, her apartment couldn't hold all the people who wanted to try this approach, and Nidetch turned the program into a new company she called Weight Watchers. The first office opened a few miles from her apartment. Forty years later, there are Weight Watchers branches in 30 countries.

THAT IS PRETTY MUCH the official history of Weight Watchers. And yes, as we'll see, Nidetch was indeed onto something when she recognized that groups could be powerful weapons in behavior change. Weight Watchers today holds more than 50,000 meetings every week at its centers, each one promoting a direct descendant of the Prudent Diet and Nidetch's program.

But there's another Weight Watchers story. This one starts in the late

1990s and involves another aspect of the company's approach to weight loss. And it looks like this:

$$p = (c \div 50) + (f \div 12) - (r \div 5)$$

This is the formula behind the Weight Watchers Points system. Though it's not exactly a secret—it's visible as part of Patent 6040531 at the US Patent and Trademark Office, though the company has tweaked it since then—the Points system is the unheralded partner in Weight Watchers' continued success. The Points system allows Weight Watchers to spread beyond groups sharing stories and provides a quantitative methodology for weight loss, treating food as an easily monitored data stream.

Though it looks intimidating at first, the Points formula is fairly straightforward, and not too far removed from Dr. Jolliffe's original strategy for weight loss. It's based on the same principle of calorie restriction: Run just enough of a calorie deficit to get the body to burn fat instead of storing it. Rather than counting calories, though, Weight Watchers members count points (the "p" in the formula) by inserting the values listed on packaged foods' Nutrition Facts labels into an equation that results in one simple number. The formula accounts not just for the calorie content of a food (the "c" in the formula) but also for the fat

The Weight Watchers Points Formula

The Points system converts the Nutrition Facts labels on food products into one simple number that lets people track how much food they consume every day.

p = number of points
c = amount of energy in calories
f = amount of fat in grams
r = amount of dietary fiber in grams

$$p = \left[\frac{c}{50}\right] + \left[\frac{f}{12}\right] - \left[\frac{r}{5}\right]$$

content (the "f") and the fiber (the "r"). Each member is allotted a certain number of points a day, depending on his or her goals and current height and weight. A typical woman gets an allowance of about 24 points per day, while the typical male is permitted about 30 points per day. In addition, members are granted 35 "flex points" each week, a splurge account they can tap into whenever the occasion or temptation arises.

The Points system was created in the late 1990s, when food conglomerate H. J. Heinz owned Weight Watchers (the company is now an independent, publicly owned company with its stock traded on the New York Stock Exchange). The timing was in many ways perfect. In the late 1990s the diet industry was in the dumps, with commercial programs like Weight Watchers and Jenny Craig and Nutrisystem all seemingly of a piece, offering twists on fad plans that, even if they worked in the short term, never took for the long term. Compared with the clinical promise of new pharmaceutical treatments like the potent fen-phen combination (which would soon be pulled from the market in 1997 when evidence emerged that it could damage heart valves and lungs), commercial weight-loss plans seemed little more than expensive gimmicks, Weight Watchers included. It didn't help that, as part of Heinz, Weight Watchers had spawned a line of foods and supplements that seemed more about pushing people to buy products than helping them lose weight.

So when the Points system arrived, it immediately offered something different. It gives members one simple target, one number that lets them track their food consumption without obsessing over it, or at least without obsessing over calories, calories, calories.

That method—turning a meal into a number—may seem fairly clinical. But it's also a way to lend some precision to deciding what you should and shouldn't eat. The Points system frames the decision in clear, specific terms. And in that precision there is control. As Weight Watchers chief scientific officer Karen Miller-Kovach, RD, says, "Points offers a system that creates a structure for people until that structure becomes habit."

And here's the thing: The Points system works, and it works on two levels. Not only does the program result in weight loss, but significantly, it's also actually a program that people will follow. Two studies published over the past decade show that the Weight Watchers plan is a far more effective way to help people lose weight—and keep it off—than willpower alone. A 2003 study published in *JAMA, the Journal of the American Medical Association,* found that nearly 40 percent of a group following the Weight Watchers program lost more than 5 percent of their body weight, almost double the success rate of a comparison group trying to lose weight on their own. What's more, the Weight Watchers group successfully kept the weight off, weighing an average of 6 pounds less more than 2 years after the study began. In other words, there's something about the system that convinces people to actually change their behavior.

A subsequent study, published in the *Annals of Internal Medicine* in 2005, gave further credence to the Weight Watchers approach. The scientific review compared the nine most popular diet programs in the United States, including Weight Watchers, Jenny Craig, eDiets.com, and Overeaters Anonymous. The review found very little scientific grounding for most commercial weight-loss programs but noted that Weight Watchers was an exception. Significantly, Weight Watchers met the benchmark of its members maintaining a 5 percent loss of their initial weight, which, the study authors wrote, "may be sufficient to prevent or ameliorate weight-related health complications."

Five percent may seem like a slight improvement, and it's hardly the transformation most people have in mind when they go on a diet. When you're starting at 200 pounds, a 5 percent loss amounts to just 10 pounds; if you weigh in at 250 pounds, a 5 percent loss translates to only 12½ pounds. But physiologically, a 5 percent loss creates real and measurable improvements in health. Lose 5 percent of your body weight, and your blood pressure and cholesterol levels fall, your risk factors for diabetes—such as your insulin resistance—drop off, and your fatty liver starts to return to normal.

So Weight Watchers' Points system seems to work, and it seems to be a program that people actually follow and stick with, unlike most other commercial diet programs. The question is: Why does it work? How, exactly, does it get people to change their behavior?

II.

EAT LESS. Exercise more.

For decades, diet and exercise have been the two commandments of preventive medicine. They constitute the ultimate in early action: If you want to improve your health, and do it before it deteriorates to the point of needing drugs or surgery, changing your behavior is all you've got. That usually boils down to eating less food (and making sure the stuff you eat is healthy) and getting more exercise.

We all know this. Yet almost none of us do anything about it.

The great majority of people in industrialized nations, and Americans in particular, should change at least some of their health behaviors. A 2004 study found that barely 3 percent of Americans were following four basic healthful behaviors: not smoking, maintaining a healthy weight, eating five servings of vegetables a day, and getting some exercise. Three percent. It's the most damning statistic about public health I've ever read, and it shows how formidable behavior change is as a social problem. This recalcitrance leads directly to bad health. In a recent study by Virginia Commonwealth University in Richmond, a whopping 71 percent of people who participated in a free behavioral counseling program had at least one significant behavior-related health risk, such as obesity, physical inactivity, or tobacco or alcohol use. Flip that around and it makes your jaw drop: Barely one-quarter of Americans are living in a healthy manner.

The problem isn't getting the word out: It's pretty much inconceivable that any conscious citizen doesn't know that obesity is unhealthy or that smoking is bad for you. That these are health risks is as close to being commonsensical as it gets. But just because we know doesn't mean we're behaving better.

In other words, this isn't an information problem. This is a systems problem. The trick is to get people to act on the information—and so far, our health care system has failed to find an effective trigger to accomplish that. This is why behavior change is among the most potent but most elusive targets in all of medicine. This is why we put so much emphasis on pharmaceuticals—because it's often easier to take a pill after we've developed a problem than to change our behavior earlier. We know that breaking our old, injurious health habits—and sticking with better, new habits—may be the most beneficial of all our health choices. But they're also the most formidable decisions to adhere to. It's the great disconnect of modern life.

ONLY IT'S NOT A MODERN PROBLEM. This is, as it turns out, a very *old* problem, one that's pretty much intrinsic to our human nature. Back in 350 BC, Aristotle called this disconnect between our intentions and our actions *akrasia,* a term that describes the conflict between reason and emotion that, we being weak-willed folk, results in our frequent failure to behave in our own best interest. Aristotle was so fascinated by this inconsistency—which is usually translated as "incontinence," meaning a lack of self-control—that he devoted an entire book of his *Ethics* to it. "Merely knowing what is right does not make a person prudent," he wrote, "he must be disposed to do it too: and the incontinent man is not so disposed."

What especially flummoxed Aristotle was that people often failed not just out of ignorance or indulgence but also for reasons that they couldn't even explain. "The man who behaves incontinently does not, before he gets into this state, think he ought to act so," the philosopher wrote. "Some people deliberate and then under the influence of their feelings fail to abide by their decision."

In a way, Aristotle's book was just the first in what's become the flourishing genre of self-help. Dr. Phil may not acknowledge the debt, but the self-help industry, the world of 12-step addiction-counseling programs and Seven Habits guides to changing your life, is fundamentally concerned with *akrasia.* The insoluble nature of the problem, in fact, is what makes it such a fertile topic for advice, offering an infinite number of methods and strategies that promise to help us change our behavior for the better—to finally do what our better natures know we should. Yet the persistence of the self-help industry only proves that, for many

The Challenge of Breaking the Habit

After as many as 14 attempts to quit, no more than 50 percent of smokers manage to quit.

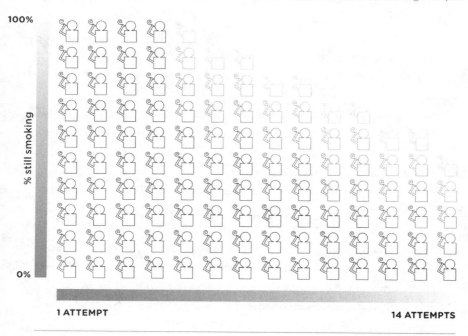

% still smoking

100%

0%

1 ATTEMPT

14 ATTEMPTS

people, none of it works. The plethora of advice, cures, and paths may make for some feel-good reads, but little of it leads to actual results.

One small comfort for those who struggle to change their unhealthy habits may be that scientists are equally baffled by the disconnect. Since the concept of health risks first emerged in the 1950s and put behavior change on the table as a viable strategy for minimizing our risks, billions of dollars have been spent on researching various strategies for getting people to change various negative behaviors. But this torrent of resources and research has yielded few true successes in terms of actionable insights into the problem. The collective conclusion of these tens of thousands of studies is that, yes, when people take steps to improve their health behaviors, they do see health benefits. But it's nearly impossible to get them to take those steps.

THIS DISCONNECT BOGGLES few people as much as it does S. Leonard Syme, PhD, an emeritus professor of epidemiology at the University of California, Berkeley, School of Public Health who's spent his career studying preventive medicine (and taught me the valuable lesson related in the Introduction). For decades, Syme has been studying populations of people for clues about how to get them to live better, from grumpy bus drivers in San Francisco, to expatriate Japanese living in Hawaii and California, to woebegone British civil servants. And in all his years of studying behavior, he's found very little that sticks, very few principles that can be disseminated as a formula for behavior change. "Behavior change is just hard," he tells me when I visit his office, and he pulls out a thick report produced by an Institute of Medicine committee he chaired not long ago. Titled *Promoting Health: Intervention Strategies from Social and Behavioral Research* and published in 2000, the book was put together "by the best people in the field," Dr. Syme says. But the report, he confesses, contains few true insights. Indeed, the recommendations—among them are more education, tougher tobacco regulation, and, above all, more research—are so banal as to be, as Dr. Syme shrugs, "worthless. Really not all that effective."

The problem, says Dr. Syme, boils down to this: "The whole field of public health is based on the idea that if we can identify the risk factors for disease and share that research with the public, they will rush home and change their behavior. That's simply not true."

Dr. Syme points to three problems with this approach. First, we have a limited understanding of the risk factors for disease in the first place. We know that poor health behaviors can lead directly to chronic diseases—diabetes, heart disease, and stroke foremost among them. And we know that most Americans—upwards of 70 percent—will die of chronic diseases. But as with the Whitehall study discussed in Chapter 1, we know too little about precisely where those connections between behavior and disease lie.

The second challenge comes down to *akrasia*. "Even when we do identify risk factors," Dr. Syme sighs, "we can't get people to change anyway." Again, Dr. Syme insists that this is not a problem of getting information to people: "People who fail to lose weight, they've tried every diet, they've read every book, they know all about what you're supposed to do. They may be experts, but they're not successful," he says.

And the third issue, says Dr. Syme, "is that even if we do get people to change their behaviors, there are always more people coming along. There always seem to be more people out there who will be developing the same risks for disease." In other words, little effort is made to stop people from entering a path that leads toward disease, and instead the emphasis is placed on helping those who are already well along the way.

Dr. Syme's favorite example of failure is the Multiple Risk Factor Intervention Trial, or MRFIT, a hugely ambitious research study that he helped design and build in the 1970s. MRFIT included about 13,000 men who had significant risks for developing coronary heart disease— they were smokers or overweight, or had high blood pressure or ate poorly, or some combination of the above. They didn't have heart disease *yet*, but if anybody was going to get it, these were the guys.

The study split them into two groups. Half were told to go to their doctors for the standard care. The other half were put through the wringer. They were taught to cook healthy meals that were low in fat and calories. They were given counseling to help them stop smoking. They were encouraged to exercise to aid in weight loss. They had frequent doctor visits to monitor their progress and encourage their compliance. And this went on for 6 years, week after week.

As hoped, those who actually followed the MRFIT protocol significantly reduced their chances of developing heart disease. But that was at best a silver lining, because most of the people failed to follow the program. Despite the counselors and classes, only 42 percent of the special case group quit smoking, and only half with high blood pressure had it under control at the end of the study. Even more disappointing, the closely monitored group showed barely any improvement in cardiac mortality over the control group.

Part of the problem, Dr. Syme surmises, was that there was something of a Hawthorne effect at work. Since the men in the control group knew they were being monitored, many of them reported that they had changed their behaviors even though they weren't being coached to do so. And another factor may have been that those in the intervention group had their behavior controlled by the trainers and the counselors. In other words, the study's structure may have let the subjects off the hook, making it so they didn't have to take control of their health on their own.

Despite its unimpressive results, MRFIT was among the first of many intensive behavior interventions over the past 40 years, many of them hugely expensive and few of them roaring successes. In the late 1990s, the Centers for Disease Control and Prevention (CDC) began its Diabetes Prevention Program (DPP), a $174 million study hoping to prove that behavioral changes can induce weight loss and prevent or delay development of type 2 diabetes. Participants in the study's lifestyle-modification arm got what resembled a sweepstakes prize: gym memberships and personal trainers, free food, and daily phone calls from nutritionists—all for 2 years or more. After all that hand-holding, those patients lost an average of 7 percent of their body weight.

At the time, the CDC hailed the DPP study as proof that diet and exercise work. True enough; as discussed above, a small change in weight can cause real metabolic improvements and lessen the risk for later disease. But really, we already knew that. And really, the gilded guidance provided by the DPP just as readily leads to a different, much less hopeful conclusion: that by doing everything for the subjects, the study didn't do much of anything for them. It failed to engage them in caring for their own health. In that case, it seems that even a relatively modest change in weight (a 7 percent weight loss by a 240-pound overweight man only brings him down to 223 pounds) requires an elaborate structure and ample resources. After all, how likely is it that the average American will stick with—let alone be able to afford—such an intensive program? It's the same reason that people on *The Biggest Loser* reality television show, while under the glare of a national TV audience and the care of professional trainers and nutritionists, lose weight—but then most of them inevitably regain the weight once they leave the show. It's difficult to change our habits for good.

And that's the larger point that a review of 40 years of behavior research shows—a point that accounts for Dr. Syme's sighs and shrugs. All of these research studies, being well designed and highly managed, take place within totally artificial environments that don't reflect reality at all. In real life, we don't have people coming into our homes, advising us on how to cook (let alone buying our food for us). Most of us don't have weekly support groups or the money for personal trainers. But most of us do have things we should do differently, bad habits that we should break—too many sodas or candy bars, too few walks or too little sleep—and if we managed to make those changes, it would lead us toward better health. More significantly, some of us have a doctor's orders to do these things: to quit smoking, or to cut out salt or fat, or to remember to take that daily aspirin. And yet in the day-to-day world, we often don't do these things. We forget. We delay. We shirk. We disobey our doctors' orders and are, as physicians say, noncompliant. Estimates of noncompliance range as high as 75 percent.

Which brings us right back to Aristotle's 2,300-year-old riddle: Why is it that people don't do what they say they will, even when they should?

III.

IN JULY 2008, APPLE COMPUTERS began allowing iPhone customers to buy small bits of software for their phones. These software programs—known as apps—allow iPhone users to do everything from play games to shop for real estate. And about half a dozen of them allow people to calculate and track their Weight Watchers Points. You just click on a food item and enter how much you ate, and the app calculates its Points value. It was easy, it was quick—and it probably violated Weight Watchers' patent.

By creating their software and selling it at Apple's app store, these independent software developers were making a buck based on somebody else's business. So that September, Weight Watchers' lawyers dispatched cease-and-desist letters to Apple and the app makers, and Apple took down the unauthorized calculators.

But a few months later, there was a new crop of Points calculators. Apple, you see, has established a robust ecosystem for app developers, making it easy for programmers to write a bit of software and sell it for a dollar or two. It's part of what makes the iPhone such a phenomenon. There are nearly 100,000 apps available, as of this writing. And while Apple does police the app store, the Points trackers are evidently too easy to create, and too easy to use, to stop altogether.

The iPhone apps didn't take Weight Watchers entirely by surprise. The company has known for several years that the Points formula has earned a passionate fan base on the Internet. Company lawyers have been sending off letters to various Web sites and software developers for years, chasing away even those who offered Points calculators for free (the formula is a terribly simple calculation for a computer). "We protect our intellectual property," says Weight Watchers CEO David Kirchhoff. "What kills us is when we have a superfan and they're putting it out there. But we can't allow people to grab snippets of our program. We have to maintain the integrity of the whole system."

Weight Watchers is undoubtedly within its rights. It's worth reminding the company, though, that the Points system itself wouldn't be possible if not for something called the Nutrition Labeling and Education Act, a bit of openness mandated by the US government in 1990 that requires all food manufacturers to state, clearly and plainly, the nutritional content of their foods. Among the quantities that must be disclosed: fat, fiber, and calories, the same three values that, with a bit of math, allow any Weight Watchers client to put the Points system to work and maybe start living a little better.

But in many ways, this is a losing battle—dozens of Points trackers are always just a Google search away. The Points system has gone viral, as they say on the Internet, and its popularity is a testament to the effectiveness of the formula. The fact that the iPhone makes this sort of app even easier to write and use will only make the Points trackers more tempting.

Put aside, for a moment, the wisdom of Weight Watchers' efforts to stop the knockoffs. Instead, let's consider what may be behind the unquenchable enthusiasm for the Points formula. The system is basic self-monitoring, or, in the language of behavioral science, an exercise in self-efficacy. Stanford psychologist Albert Bandura, PhD, coined the term "self-efficacy" in 1977 to describe his belief that individuals hold the power and resources to achieve certain goals. Self-efficacy means that we ourselves hold the keys to our lives.

Though he's far from a household name, among psychologists and behavior researchers, Dr. Bandura stands alongside Sigmund Freud for his work in explaining the mechanisms of human behavior. And just as Freud's revolutionary insights seem almost clichéd a century later (the id and the ego; the conscious and the subconscious), Dr. Bandura's work is seemingly simple, and much of what he proposed about human behavior comes across today as common sense. Dr. Bandura suggested, for instance, that in order to change behaviors such as phobias or substance abuse, people need to set specific goals and track their status and progress toward these benchmarks. Such monitoring keeps people mindful of how they're progressing, Dr. Bandura proposed. And it serves another purpose as well: "Participants acquire a generalizable skill for dealing successfully with stressful situations," he wrote, "a skill that they use to overcome a variety of dysfunctional fears and inhibitions in their everyday life." In other words, not only is self-tracking an effective way to track progress, it's also a tool that individuals can use to cope. It gives them control.

Dr. Bandura's insights about self-efficacy form the cornerstone of what has come to be known as social cognitive theory. Again, the fact that you may not have heard of it only testifies to its broad reach today. In contrast with the classic behaviorist view that our actions are specific responses to specific stimuli, Dr. Bandura's theory suggests that our behavior is the consequence of feedback from a variety of personal factors, actions, and the environment. Where classic behaviorism affords little influence to the individual, social cognitive theory proposes that the individual is presented with a powerful opportunity when reacting to this feedback stream. By tailoring the feedback that we receive to reflect specific goals, Dr. Bandura believed that we can successfully change our behavior.

Since Dr. Bandura first proposed his self-efficacy model and social cognitive theory more than 30 years ago, feedback has emerged as one of the most powerful tools for behavior change, and one of the few principles that actually help people accomplish change. The science bears Dr. Bandura out: The recently completed ALIVE (A Lifestyle Intervention Via Email) study, which hoped to improve people's diets and increase their physical activity (in other words: *eat less, exercise more*), had about 800 people track 35 physical activities in minute detail: how much they walked, how often and how intensely they played sports, how frequently they watched TV. It likewise tracked their diets across dozens of food items, by quantity, frequency, portion size, and nutritional content. Those data were used to generate individually tailored goals sent to participants via e-mail to help them stay on track. After 4 months' time, the participants were significantly more likely than a control group to have successfully changed their behavior. What's more, they were twice as likely to feel *empowered* to change their diets. The feedback wasn't just changing their health; it changed the way they thought about their health.

What's at work here? Feedback is overcoming Aristotle's *akrasia* and putting our behavior to work for us, rather than against us. This isn't information cast upon us by a disciplinarian, it's coming from within. As it happens, and fortunately so for Weight Watchers, a numbers-based feedback model suits a diet program particularly well. Nutritional information is easily quantified and monitored. Food, when you get down to it, is just an input. And that's why public health researchers are starting to believe self-tracking is not only an important tool for improving behavior but also a revolutionary one. It is, as one textbook describes it, "perhaps the single-most important ingredient to successful dietary change efforts."

FEEDBACK, THOUGH, ISN'T THE ONLY FACTOR working in Weight Watchers' favor. There's another component to the Weight Watchers strategy, one that Jean Nidetch hit upon in her living room back in the 1960s: "the magic of the meeting," as her company calls it.

The group is the one constant in the Weight Watchers plan. It is, for one thing, where the company gets a fair amount of its revenue, in the form of the $9 or so every member must pay to attend a weekly meeting. To chief scientific officer Karen Miller-Kovach, the groups serve two purposes for members: They give people a social environment in which to share and commiserate, and they keep people on track with the program, because, she says, "knowing you've got that meeting every week, and that weigh-in every week, keeps you accountable."

Group meetings, of course, are hardly a Weight Watchers invention. From Alcoholics Anonymous to Debtors Anonymous to all the other 12-step organizations, groups have long been considered a worthy tool for improving behavior. This makes perfect sense; psychology alone would argue that groups allow us to compare ourselves with others, to learn good habits and trade tricks that will help us navigate our way to better behavior.

Dr. Bandura paved the way here, too. His early research, in the 1960s, introduced the concept of modeling, in which we measure ourselves and calibrate our behavior by comparing it with that of others. Dr. Bandura demonstrated this in his famous "Bobo doll" experiments. Recruiting 72 children from the Stanford University Nursery School, Dr. Bandura had each child in the experimental group sit with an adult in a room filled with toys, the most notable being a 5-foot-tall inflatable figure known as a Bobo doll. With some children, the adult would pick up a mallet and hit the Bobo doll repeatedly. With other children, the adult would play gently with other toys. (A control group of children was put in the room without an adult present.)

After being exposed to the adult's behavior, the child was left in the room alone. As Dr. Bandura had expected, the children's behavior was strongly influenced by the adult's—those who had witnessed the adult's violent behavior were much more likely to hit the Bobo doll themselves (and male children even more so than females) than were those who hadn't been exposed to violent play.

The insight may seem obvious today, but the Bobo doll experiment allowed Dr. Bandura to isolate a particularly important concept:

Behavior isn't entirely innate. We are likely to be influenced by the behavior of others; indeed, behavior can in some regard be modified. It's the concept that's undergirded most of the science investigating group dynamics ever since.

In recent years, there's been a growing effort to measure the power of group dynamics for changing behavior. In the 1990s, the Project Active study compared people who exercised in supervised groups to those who tried to increase their activity independently. The study found that the people in the groups had much more success (in terms of weight loss and overall fitness gains) than those working alone. Other studies have also supported groups as effective tools for change. The problem, though, is that group programs—at least as they're conceived of in research studies—can be expensive. Certainly, it's beyond many people's means to participate in a program that offers regular meetings, one-on-one counseling, and constant monitoring.

But another body of evidence is emerging that says that groups needn't be so highly structured to yield benefits. Nicholas Christakis, MD, PhD, a sociologist and physician at Harvard Medical School, and James Fowler, PhD, a political scientist at the University of California, San Diego, have spent the past several years examining how social networks can magnify health effects even when they're not designed to do so. Using data from the Framingham Heart Study, Dr. Christakis and Dr. Fowler studied the smoking habits of 12,000 people, looking for correlations between their smoking status and their social relationships. The results, published in 2008 in the *New England Journal of Medicine*, showed quite clearly that relationships greatly influenced whether people smoked—and whether they succeeded at quitting. In fact, it seemed that people successfully stopped smoking when entire clusters quit almost in concert. If your sibling also quit, you were 25 percent more likely to succeed yourself, and if your wife or husband also quit, you were 67 percent more likely to quit. The same held true with co-workers and friends (34 percent and 36 percent, respectively). "Because people are connected, their health is connected," explains Dr. Christakis. "Social networks tend to magnify whatever they are seeded with."

What was at play among the smokers in Framingham? Since this

How to Quit Smoking

Stopping smoking isn't just hard because it's an addiction—it's also difficult because there are so many ways to try to quit. And considering how difficult it is to break the habit, maybe that's a good thing.

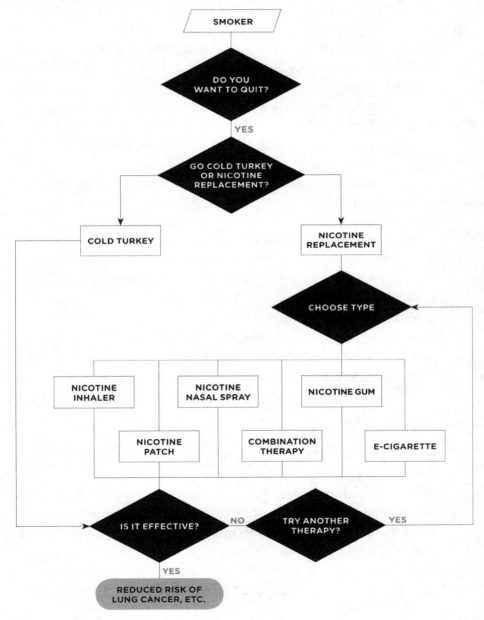

was a data analysis, not an intervention study, there was no artificial, expensive experiment going on. This was purely a social phenomenon— a demonstration of what is called a network effect. This is what's at work when something "goes viral" on the Web, or when you have the same joke e-mailed to you by all your friends on the same day. The fact that this can compel people to stop smoking, almost spontaneously, is a powerful testament to the power of groups, and a potential tool in driving behavior change. As Dr. Christakis says, "Our current understanding of health is very incomplete. It's focused too narrowly on the individual level. But there are external components of individual health. To really understand individual health, we have to understand how groups work. We have to understand community."

Dr. Christakis and Dr. Fowler have also shown that social networks can be powerful contributors to *bad* behavior as well. Another analysis they did of the Framingham data tracked obesity through the network and found that it, too, spread like a virus. If someone had a friend who became obese, that person's chances of following suit increased by 57 percent. Dr. Christakis's hypothesis is that as friends and family grew obese, the stigma around the condition lessened.

What Weight Watchers has hit on, then, is an especially powerful combination of quantified feedback and social networks. This combination transforms a group from a collective "shoulder to cry on" into a tool of science. The group becomes a comparative, cooperative, and even competitive arena that can lead to better decisions.

BUT WAIT. If Dr. Bandura identified this stuff 30 years ago and Weight Watchers has been exploiting these ideas for a decade, then what's the mystery about behavior change? Why haven't that knowledge and all that research solved this problem years ago? Why aren't we inundated with self-tracking tools and groups at every turn? Why is this still Weight Watchers' secret? Or, to put it another way: If we already know this, then why are people still so fat?

The answer is that, until recently, though the principles have been well known, the tools to turn them into action have not been well distributed. It's hard—often too hard—to get people to adopt the feedback and groups that will help them get started. Food journals and exercise logs and drug diaries are all attempts to create feedback loops. But they fail because they tack an additional behavior on top of the ones we're trying to introduce or change; they require us to remember to pick up the pen and fill out the chart. And then, having charted our progress, we have to assess it and consider what it tells us. These are all extra steps, and that extra effort makes feedback more difficult to come by. In other words, it requires two levels of compliance: first, a commitment to behave differently, and then a *further* commitment to track and monitor our behavior. This extra step is, for most people, just enough of an obstacle to make feedback difficult to obtain. The same thing goes for groups: It's difficult to get people to haul themselves to a meeting room every week, especially when they're people with bad habits to begin with. It takes motivation to leave home to get motivated.

This has been the paradox of behavior change: People have to adopt new behaviors in order to change bad behaviors. And these extra levels of work mean that Dr. Bandura's principles are often cited but more often neglected. What we need, then, is a way to make it easier for people to track their behavior, a way to make it easier for people to gather in groups. What we need is a catalyst, a mechanism. And now we have one. It's called the Internet.

It turns out that the Internet is especially good at facilitating both of these principles for behavior change, but we know them by different names. In the world of information technology, the word for feedback is *data,* and the term for group support is *social network.* More than perhaps any other factor, data and social networks are the two ingredients that have made the Internet such a revolutionary force in our culture over the past 15 years. The World Wide Web, after all, was built as a way to share information among people of common interests—to make it easy to enter data, manipulate it, discuss it, and learn from it. The Internet is an information system. Think about how Google has changed your life and the way you retrieve and use information. The Internet is likewise a social network, a web that easily connects people with similar interests without regard for time or geography. Think about how Facebook has changed the way you communicate with friends.

These, of course, are the very principles of early action, data, and openness that underlie the science of a Decision Tree. This is ideal ground for behavior change: a chance to combine the behavioral theorist's principles of feedback and group communication with the technologist's tools of data and social networks. These are, when it comes down to it, the *same things*. The opportunity we have at hand is to take advantage of the fact that science and technology have arrived at the same point at nearly the same time. If it's well demonstrated that the Internet is the greatest tool for information and collaboration in history, then it follows that it could be just as significant a tool for behavior change as well.

IV.

IN LATE OCTOBER 2007, 3,410 women lined up on a starting line and ran a race together without ever seeing a glimpse of each other. They weren't running at night. They were running in the first Nike+ virtual half-marathon, each of them wearing a sensor that tracked her speed and distance. Though these women were running in different cities, they all started at the same time and ran the official half-marathon distance of exactly 13.1 miles. It was an unprecedented experiment in community and data gathering, one that was one-upped a year later when 1 million people worldwide used their Nike+ sensors to run a 10-K race in 25 cities around the world. Called the Human Race, it was the biggest participatory sporting event in world history.

The Nike+ sensor consists of just three parts: There's an accelerometer that detects when your foot hits and leaves the ground, calculating your distance. There's a transmitter that sends the information to a receiver connected to an Apple iPod. And there's the battery. That's what Nike+ is.

What's more interesting is what Nike+ isn't. There's no global positioning system (GPS) that automatically tracks your route; if you want to map your run, you have to do it manually on the Nike site. There's no heart-rate monitor, so even though you know how far and how fast you've traveled, you don't know what level of cardiovascular exertion it required. "We really wanted to separate ourselves from that sort of very technical, geeky side of things," says Michael Tchao, who helped develop the product at Nike. "Everyone understands speed and distance."

In other words, Nike+ doesn't measure everything one could imagine measuring; it wasn't designed to. But it's good enough, and, more crucially, it's simple. Nike learned a huge lesson from Apple: The iPod wasn't a massive hit because it was the most powerful music player on the market, but because it offered the easiest, most streamlined user experience. So far, more than 1.2 million runners have tracked more than 130 million miles and burned more than 13 billion calories.

All that data gets sent to the Nike+ Web site (http://nikerunning. nike.com/nikeplus), where runners can share and compare their results. They can join teams and set group workout goals. And they can announce open challenges, plotting virtual routes that any runner on the Nike+ system can follow. (This lets runners in New York City, for instance, take a trek across Canada just by running laps around the Central Park reservoir.)

That wealth of data can lead to novel insights: The most popular day for running is Sunday, and most Nike+ users tend to work out in the evening. After the holidays, there's a huge increase in the number of goals that runners set; in January 2009, they set three times as many goals as the month before. And Nike has discovered that there's a magic number for a Nike+ user: five. If someone uploads only a couple of runs to the site, they might just be trying it out. But once they hit five runs, they're massively more likely to keep running and uploading data. At five runs, they're hooked on what their data tell them about themselves.

Though the Nike+ system started as a device for avid runners, it has broad appeal among people who find that tracking their movement—specifically, the calories-burned estimates—can provide incentive for doing other exercise, too. Walkers have taken to using Nike+ for lower-intensity exercise. And those who find running tedious can download soundtracks for data-driven aerobic workouts at Apple's iTunes store.

The Nike+ online forums are chock-full of people who praise the system for helping them lose weight, and thousands of Nike+-equipped bloggers are tracking their weight-loss progress in public. "It just made running so much more entertaining for me," says Veronica Noone, who blogs at ronisweigh.com and has used Nike+ to go from 210 to 145 pounds. "There's something about seeing what you've done, how your pace changes as you go up and down hills, that made me more motivated."

Nike+ is just one of dozens of gadgets geared toward the exercise and weight-loss markets, and more are popping up every day. The fitbit is a $99 gizmo that lets you track daily movement, calorie consumption, and sleep quality. Some cell phones now come with built-in GPS sensors and accelerometers that let you track your movements and exercise. Nintendo's Wii video game console, which uses an accelerometer with a gyro sensor to track movement, has Wii Fit, a package that turns exercise into a video game by tracking your weight and the calories you burn as you bounce and shake around your living room. These and several other services work the nexus between tracking activity and changing behavior.

So how is it that a shoe company and a weight-loss company have managed to create popular and effective tools for behavior change while medical professionals still shrug at the problem of rising obesity rates? What do Nike and Weight Watchers know that medicine doesn't? The answer, it turns out, may not matter. These companies may or may not be aware of the science behind their tools (in the case of Nike, they seem to have stumbled upon behavior change rather than aimed for it; in the case of Weight Watchers, they started with someone else's science and created their own research after the fact). The fact is that they're available now and the public is responding.

Indeed, traditional science is the laggard here, because it takes years for researchers to examine these technologies and assess their effectiveness. By using the very principles that health behavior research has established—personalized information is more effective than generalized information, as is setting clear goals and then incremental goals within them—Nike+ and its ilk are far ahead of anything the medical community has come up with.

Putting these principles to work in an online environment doesn't just make them easier, it makes them emphatically more effective. Weight Watchers, it turns out, knows that the combination is an especially potent one; the company's internal research shows that members who use the Web site in conjunction with going to the meetings and using the Points system have 50 percent greater weight loss than those who only use the program offline.

In late 2009, after a year of cease-and-desist letters and efforts to quash the unauthorized iPhone Points trackers, Weight Watchers released its own app for the iPhone. It lets people count Points and track their progress. David Kirchhoff, Weight Watchers' CEO, has great hopes for the Points app. But he insists that its success will be measured, ultimately, by how well it helps people meet their goals. "There are 20 to 25 habit changes that people need to accomplish in order to lose weight. It takes a long time and a lot of work to get there. There's no magic in it. Tracking is just good science. And sharing our experiences and being open about our experiences, that can ultimately slay the demon."

PART II

Diagnosis and Detection

No Such Thing as Normal

How Risk for Disease Became a Disease All Its Own

I.

CAROL NELSON KNEW SHE WASN'T IN GREAT HEALTH. Years ago, she'd gained 60 pounds during a pregnancy. Now, Carol (her name has been changed, but the details of her story are true) found herself stuck at more than 220 pounds. And the weight was just the start of it. She always felt fatigued, and her hands and feet were often swollen. She wasn't sick so much as just *unwell*.

Over the years, various specialists (rheumatologists, endocrinologists, internists) had offered various diagnoses (high blood pressure, hypothyroidism, osteoarthritis) and prescribed various medications (levothyroxine, celecoxib). But nothing worked. "I was really at the end of my rope, really thought whatever I had was going to kill me," she says. "And it would have, had I not found out what the problem was. You can't fight an enemy when you don't know who he is."

The breakthrough came when a new endocrinologist diagnosed her with something called metabolic syndrome. She'd never heard of it. But as she Googled and learned more, her chronic ailments—the weight, the high blood pressure, the lack of energy—started to make sense. They even seemed treatable. Carol went on metformin and rosiglitazone (both of which regulate blood sugar), and she lost 20 pounds by cutting out carbohydrates. And she started to feel less sick. She started to feel better. "Getting a diagnosis was a relief," she says. "I have hope now, whereas I didn't have any before."

Carol Nelson is among the first wave of people to be diagnosed with metabolic syndrome, a condition that, though concretely defined only 8 years ago, is now said to afflict about 25 percent of American adults. The disease is rife worldwide: In Ireland, 20 percent of adults meet the disease criteria, and in India, an incredible 40 percent of adults could be diagnosed with the syndrome. We sit, indeed, amid an epidemic of metabolic syndrome, a fact all the more remarkable because so few people are familiar with it. For this is no virus on the loose, no plague that has spread unchecked. Rather, metabolic syndrome is just a new way to think about a cluster of well-known and increasingly prevalent conditions. Metabolic syndrome is characterized by five risk factors: high blood pressure, high blood sugar, high triglycerides (fatty acids in the bloodstream), low HDL ("good") cholesterol, and obesity. Of the five, obesity is the most important, because the rise in the numbers of the morbidly overweight is directly driving the rise in the syndrome. Metabolic syndrome is, in fact, almost indistinguishable from obesity—at least 85 percent of those who have the syndrome are obese or overweight.

But is it real? In some ways, no. Since it's a checklist of risk factors rather than symptoms, it stretches the way we think of disease. It's very much a human invention, a "syndrome"—the term researchers assign to things they don't quite understand. But in other ways, it's absolutely real. Though championed by drug companies, it's also been defined and recognized by legitimate health organizations. And having it is definitely unhealthy. You can't die of metabolic syndrome, but you can die of what it leads to: diabetes and heart disease.

The ambiguity surrounding metabolic syndrome has made it a controversial diagnosis in the medical community. Critics say that metabolic syndrome lumps together risks we already recognize and monitor. Worse, some say that it's just a fancy way to describe obesity. By accepting it, they say, we turn a lifestyle problem into a medical problem. After all, the treatment for metabolic syndrome is the same as that for

Carol Nelson's Decision Tree

Carol Nelson went through lots of doctors and diagnoses before being told she had metabolic syndrome, a risk-based condition that can lead to diabetes or heart disease. It was just what she needed to make some changes in her life.

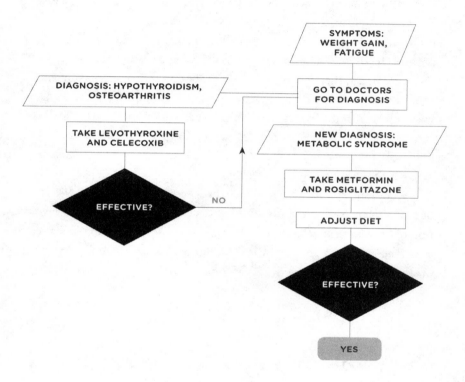

SYMPTOMS: WEIGHT GAIN, FATIGUE

DIAGNOSIS: HYPOTHYROIDISM, OSTEOARTHRITIS

GO TO DOCTORS FOR DIAGNOSIS

TAKE LEVOTHYROXINE AND CELECOXIB

NEW DIAGNOSIS: METABOLIC SYNDROME

EFFECTIVE?

NO

TAKE METFORMIN AND ROSIGLITAZONE

ADJUST DIET

EFFECTIVE?

YES

obesity and many other poor-lifestyle conditions: diet and exercise.

The debate surrounding metabolic syndrome is, in many respects, a consequence of the increase in risk-based diagnoses in medicine. These conditions exist not because they are themselves deadly, but because they're harbingers of worse conditions likely to come later. For people like Carol Nelson, getting a diagnosis of metabolic syndrome might be a useful way to engage with their health, to get serious about it. Doing so is quite clearly based on the principles of using data and acting early. On the other hand, the "emergence" of metabolic syndrome is symptomatic of how disease-centric our health care has become. If we don't engage with our health until we get sick, well then, maybe it's best if anybody can be classified as sick. And in that sense, the syndrome assigning seems like a cop-out, a way of giving people a diagnosis simply because their lifestyles have gotten away from them.

Metabolic syndrome, in other words, could be the great disease of our age. Or it could be a sign of how diseased our age is, a demonstration of how certain we are that there is always a scientific explanation, a diagnosis, and perhaps a pill for what ails us. Either way, metabolic syndrome is a disease whose time has come.

II.

THESE DAYS, TREATING RISK is a well-established principle in medicine. We treat high cholesterol because it is associated with a greater risk of developing heart disease. We treat high blood pressure, or, as the more medically minded call it, hypertension, because it carries a higher risk of stroke. We even treat something called subdiabetic hyperglycemia, formerly known as prediabetes, because it carries a risk of leading to (you guessed it) diabetes.

This bevy of risk-based conditions stems largely from two principles. The great upsurge of chronic disease in the developed world has compelled the fields of public health and medicine to try to identify the precursors of disease, such as was done in the Framingham study and other research efforts. Risk goes hand in hand with chronic disease—a "disease of civilization" that medicine was, at first, poorly prepared to fight. Only by codifying the risks that led to these diseases did medicine finally begin to counter the tide of chronic disease.

Second, the move to identify risk-based conditions results from physicians' "treat the numbers" approach to health care. More careful tests and measurements of various factors—blood pressure, cholesterol, blood glucose—have allowed physicians to assess our health well before we ourselves may feel a symptom. This becomes a numbers game, with doctors trying to move certain numbers down or up and prescribing treatments accordingly. In the main, this is beneficial and good. It gets us thinking about our health before we otherwise might. But it also changes the way we think about health and illness.

Indeed, these days we judge our doctors not just by how well they cure us of disease, but by how adequately they identify the precursors of diseases in order to get a jump on treatment. Millions of Americans take aspirin every day not for headaches but to prevent heart attacks, while millions more are prescribed statin drugs that lower their cholesterol. We get these prescriptions and take these pills almost without a second thought, as if we are treating disease, not just a risk of disease.

It wasn't always so. Just a few decades back, the connection between disease and risk was poorly understood, even for the most common fatal conditions, like heart disease and cancer. And though numbers may have been at hand, there was no method for responding to them if symptoms didn't present themselves.

Take the case of Franklin Delano Roosevelt. In 1931, 14 years before he would die of a stroke and a year before he was elected to his first term as president, FDR had a blood pressure of 140 over 100. The 140—Roosevelt's systolic reading, indicating the peak pressure of blood in his arteries each time his heart beat—would today be classified as stage 1 hypertension. But the diastolic reading of 100—which indicates the minimum pressure in his arteries, between heartbeats—is by today's standards clearly in the range of stage 2, or moderately high, hypertension, high enough so that most physicians would begin therapy with medication.

But in 1931, doctors didn't know that. This was still 17 years before the Framingham study of heart disease began, and decades before there was a clear course of treatment for hypertension. So nothing was done for FDR's condition, even as the numbers ticked upward year after year. By 1937, when Roosevelt began his second term, his blood pressure had worsened to 169 over 98, with his systolic reading entering what is now a clear danger zone. By 1941, it had reached 188 over 105. And in 1944, his reading was 210 over 120, numbers that would send you straight to the hospital today. But at the time, Roosevelt's personal physician wrote simply that the president showed "a moderate degree of arteriosclerosis, although no more than normal for a man of his age."

By February of 1945, FDR's blood pressure stood at 260 over 150, a level that physicians now term malignant hypertension, an emergency condition in which the kidneys are in danger of shutting down. And yet, with World War II winding down, Roosevelt continued to make international diplomatic trips, and he continued to smoke (this was years before the dangers of smoking became known as well). He was prescribed phenobarbital, a sedative. And on April 12 of that year, President Roosevelt died of a massive stroke. His physician said that it "had come out of the clear sky."

Today, it's unthinkable that anybody in Roosevelt's condition, with his access to the best health care available, could decline so dramatically without intervention or treatment. But at the time, just more than 60 years ago, hypertension was only beginning to emerge as a condition that, in and of itself, deserved to be treated. His doctors may have been tracking FDR's numbers, but they weren't treating them. Without a physical symptom—headache, nausea, palpitations, fainting—there was no evidence that could lead to a valid diagnosis. The blood pressure data were useless if they weren't backed up by something the doctors could actually see with their eyes. Indeed, some physicians at the time believed high blood pressure was an "important compensatory mechanism" that indicated that the body was trying to fix itself.

With the beginning of the Framingham Heart Study and the expansion of the National Institutes of Health in the late 1940s, preventing disease became a national priority in the United States, and identifying and treating risk became a fundamental tool of medicine. Hypertension was the obvious test case here, since blood pressure is easily measured and, thanks to Framingham, clearly associated with heart disease and death. In the 1950s, antihypertensive medications began to appear, drugs that reduced blood pressure and, in turn, decreased one's chances of developing heart disease or having a heart attack. The most popular of these was Diuril (chlorothiazide), which Merck released in 1959.

Indeed, Diuril so effectively lowered blood pressure that doctors found themselves in a quandary. If a patient was found to have high blood pressure but no other symptoms of illness, a physician could conceivably begin treatment based on the blood pressure reading alone. For physicians, who at that time were trained to diagnose a disease only when symptoms appeared, this was a wholly unexpected approach to their craft. At first, many physicians rejected the idea; in a sublimely clinical coinage, one doctor argued that high blood pressure was "not a true but a sphygmomanometric disease," referring to the sphygmomanometer, the technical name for a blood pressure monitor. By the end of the 1960s, though, this debate had effectively ended, as a definitive study of war veterans showed that treating hypertension with Diuril had a significant effect in preventing further complications. The study helped establish the now-common 120 over 80 ceiling for normal blood pressure. Treating the numbers became the norm.

By the time the word *hypercholesterolemia* began to turn up regularly in research papers in the 1960s and 1970s, the idea of risk-based disease was well established. The argument for fighting high cholesterol, however, was a bit more complicated than that for high blood pressure. Unlike hypertension, which research had identified as a dangerous if invisible condition, high cholesterol had only been *associated* with later heart disease. At best, high cholesterol seemed to be a red flag, an indication of risk, but not an indication that suggested the need for a specific treatment. That distinction was essential, because whereas treating high blood pressure helped to save lives, there was no similar evidence that treating high cholesterol would actually reduce the risk of heart disease. As late as 1980, the National Academy of Sciences was suggesting that treating cholesterol was unjustified, given the research.

It wasn't until the development of statin drugs in the late 1980s that lowering high cholesterol could be clearly connected with preventing cardiovascular disease. This research shifted the conversation on cholesterol, establishing it alongside high blood pressure as an obvious precursor of disease that must be treated as a disease in and of itself. About 33 million Americans are or should be on statin drugs, based on the current recommendations (the cutoff for treatment has dropped over the years from 300 milligrams of total cholesterol per deciliter to 260 to 240 to 200 to, as of this writing, 180). It's among the largest categories of pharmaceuticals, bringing in tens of billions of dollars in revenue for drug companies. And more than 2 decades after their arrival, the enthusiasm for statins is only increasing: Nearly every month, a new study shows that the drugs reduce risk not just of heart disease but also of stroke, macular degeneration, even asthma. Each such study potentially expands the market for the drugs; citing growing research, cardiologists at Johns Hopkins University in Baltimore in 2009 recommended further lowering the cutoff for statin prescription to pull in as many as 6.5 million more Americans. The aggregate effect isn't just the expansion of one condition. It expands the concept of risk itself. Combine the number of people taking statins for cholesterol with the number taking ACE inhibitors for high blood pressure or rosiglitazone for prediabetes, and "risk" becomes a disease unto itself. No other term brings so many people to medical treatment (at so great a return) as does risk.

III.

SCOTT GRUNDY, MD, PHD, is the Billy Graham of metabolic syndrome. The director of the Center for Human Nutrition at the University of Texas Southwestern Medical Center in Dallas, Dr. Grundy is often on the dais, spreading the good word. Turn up at a meeting like the Metabolic Diseases Drug Discovery and Development World Summit; or the Obesity, Lifestyle, and Cardiovascular Disease Symposium; or the Targeting Metabolic Syndrome conference, and odds are that Dr. Grundy is on the program.

"What we see in patients with metabolic syndrome is a two- to threefold increase in risk for developing cardiovascular disease," he told a Washington, DC, audience a few years ago in his standard stump speech. "If all of the patients who have this syndrome are at high lifetime risk for both [cardiovascular disease] and diabetes, it is important to identify such patients as early as possible."

He's been evangelizing like this since 2001, when he took up the chairmanship of the National Cholesterol Education Campaign (NCEC). In treatment guidelines known as the Adult Treatment Panel III, or ATP III, issued in 2001 and updated in 2004, Dr. Grundy and his NCEC colleagues called out metabolic syndrome as a condition that "is as strong a contributor to early heart disease as cigarette smoking." It was a remarkable statement, considering how established the risk from cigarettes was and how few in the medical community had even heard of metabolic syndrome.

The ATP III codified what had been a largely academic term into a new and suddenly dangerous clinical diagnosis. With a bit of math, it became clear that metabolic syndrome was nearly ubiquitous, with as many as 50 million Americans fitting under its diagnostic umbrella (as the definition was tweaked, the number would climb to 75 million by 2010). People with the syndrome are twice as likely to die from—and three times as likely to have—a heart attack or stroke as people without it, according to the International Diabetes Federation. It's a disease more prevalent than arthritis and asthma combined.

The ATP III kick-started the metabolic syndrome machine. The World Health Organization assigned it an International Classification of Diseases code, a crucial step that let physicians diagnose it and refer to it in insurance documents. Conferences, research studies, and drug development followed. "A few things came together," Dr. Grundy told me. "One, metabolic syndrome was becoming very common; with the rise in obesity, we've seen a rise in all these risk factors. Two, the drug companies saw an opportunity for new drug development, to see if they could target several things at once. So obesity is driving the syndrome, and also driving interest in the syndrome."

Dr. Grundy was already a recognized pioneer in heart disease and cholesterol research by the time the ATP III report came out. In the 1990s, he spearheaded the research that proved that statin drugs lower cholesterol levels. With metabolic syndrome, he's writing another chapter in his autobiography. Over the past decade, he has written or coauthored more than 100 papers on obesity and metabolic syndrome.

To Dr. Grundy, the connection between obesity and metabolic syndrome is inextricable—one leads to the other, and they both lead to an increased risk of an early death. Given that obesity is the most pressing public health issue of our day, Dr. Grundy says, the rise of metabolic syndrome should be setting off alarms. "Have you ever been to the Orlando airport? Taken a look at the size of those people? This isn't going away." These are the people, he adds, who are most likely to develop diabetes (the number with the disease in the United States has almost doubled in the past decade, nearly all due to obesity), and they are more likely to die of heart disease than those who aren't overweight. Boosting awareness of the syndrome, Dr. Grundy believes, may be our best chance to defuse this time bomb.

Not everyone in the medical community, however, has jumped on the bandwagon. In 2003, Richard Kahn, PhD, chief scientific and medical officer for the American Diabetes Association (ADA) at the time, began looking into metabolic syndrome. He reviewed 5 years of research—some 10,000 papers in all—to assess whether the diagnosis had any measurable clinical value. Was the syndrome, he wondered, a better indicator of long-term risk than any of the individual risks? Did diagnosing metabolic syndrome actually improve rates of heart disease and diabetes? In other words, was the sum of the cutoffs and checklist of conditions greater than its parts?

Dr. Kahn's results, published in September 2005 as a joint statement from the ADA and the European Association for the Study of Diabetes, stunned the medical establishment: He found no proof that a diagnosis of metabolic syndrome better predicted long-term cardiovascular disease. "Our analysis indicates that too much critically important information is missing to warrant its designation as a 'syndrome,' " Dr. Kahn and his coauthors wrote. "Until much-needed research is completed, clinicians should evaluate and treat all [cardiovascular disease] risk factors without regard to whether a patient meets the criteria for diagnosis of the 'metabolic syndrome'."

Dr. Kahn is a skeptic by nature. He doesn't disagree that considering and modifying risk factors are essential components of treating disease and of reducing the number of people who get a disease in the first place. He is quite proud, for instance, of the diabetes risk calculator that the ADA has set up on its Web site that will rate your chances of developing diabetes. But he is concerned that, with metabolic syndrome, there is a tendency to flag a risk that doesn't meaningfully connect to whether people's lives will be improved. "It became codified into an explicit disease, and then the train left the station. But the definition is arbitrary, it's pulled out of the air," he says. "As a way of saying you're at risk for something, it's a very poor predictor."

And yet, for Carol Nelson and thousands like her, terminology matters. There's something about taking high blood pressure and obesity and calling it metabolic syndrome that makes it different—even if it's unclear what that difference is. Likewise for physicians. In a doctor's office, Dr. Grundy says, "physicians see a patient with diabetes or hyperglycemia and they focus so much on that, there is a real danger they will ignore blood pressure or lipids. It becomes tunnel vision. By saying that these all go together as metabolic syndrome, some of us believe it leads doctors to look at the whole patient and this patient's total risk."

IV.

DR. KAHN IS RIGHT ABOUT ONE THING: The definition of metabolic syndrome is an exercise in idiosyncrasy. Since 1999, no fewer than 10 different sets of numbers have been proposed to define and diagnose the syndrome. Most of these definitions agree on the big points: that the syndrome is a confluence of obesity and high blood sugar, high cholesterol, high triglycerides, and high blood pressure. But each of these definitions uses slightly different numbers and cutoffs. And this raises some questions, starting with the basic ones: Where do the numbers come from? Who decides what they are and when to change them?

Here are the five criteria that the American Heart Association, under advisement from Dr. Grundy, stands by at the time of this writing:

- Elevated waist circumference: for men, equal to or greater than 40 inches; for women, equal to or greater than 35 inches
- Elevated triglycerides: equal to or greater than 150 milligrams per deciliter (mg/dl)
- Reduced HDL cholesterol: for men, less than 40 mg/dl; for women, less than 50 mg/dl
- Elevated blood pressure: equal to or greater than 130/85 millimeters of mercury (mmHg), or use of medication for hypertension
- Elevated fasting glucose: equal to or greater than 100 mg/dl

Don't worry if all those numbers make your eyes glaze over. Many doctors feel the same way. As Dr. Kahn argues, this profusion of criteria and almost random collection of data points—waist size!—makes the syndrome a rather murky condition. To Dr. Kahn, all the precision is illusory, little more than hand waving to distract us from the fiction behind the syndrome. But on the other hand, these metrics offer a concrete way to understand disease. There's a certain clarity to it; it is precise and quantitative, and it's also fairly straightforward. Given a tape measure, a blood pressure monitor, and a routine blood test, any of us could diagnose it in ourselves.

The fact is that the apparent arbitrariness of how metabolic syndrome is defined—and the similar arbitrariness in defining other diseases by metrics and cutoffs, from vitamin deficiencies to Cushing's syndrome to hyperparathyroidism—is what happens when we try to anticipate disease rather than wait for it, when we choose to define disease rather than be defined by it. The further we move away from symptom-based diagnosis, the more we depend on benchmarks and cutoff points to define disease and confirm a diagnosis.

But it makes the idea of disease—and of health, for that matter—an abstraction. Thresholds are lowered, classifying ever greater numbers of people as "diseased," in a phenomenon that's happened not just with metabolic syndrome but also with diabetes, osteoporosis, hypertension, and high cholesterol. As the definitions and benchmarks and cutoffs change, millions of people who were defined as healthy can be suddenly reclassified as unhealthy. One estimate suggests that new definitions for high cholesterol, hypertension, diabetes, and overweight lump 75 percent of American adults into the category of those having chronic diseases.

That, of course, is the demographic ripple effect that happens with diseases like metabolic syndrome. As the medical establishment reaches further down the causal chain to identify more risk factors and spot them earlier, and as it assigns names, definitions, and treatments to these diagnoses, more and more people are swept up in the net. Add in our genetic biomarkers and it's clear that disease won't be something we can avoid anymore. It will be something we simply have, just as we have freckles or wear glasses. We all will carry our disease portfolios and be identified through our ailments—or, more precisely, through our inclinations toward certain ailments. Metabolic syndrome is just the latest step on this path.

On one level, this is the inevitable progress of medicine. Identifying risks for disease has saved millions of lives. But it's a subtly different matter when the objective shifts from identifying *risks* earlier to creating *diseases* based on an assemblage of risks. Taken to its extreme, this further step makes the idea of disease—and of health, for that matter—a condition that we can never really discern. "We all already have a disease," Dr. Kahn told me one afternoon. "Life: It's a terminal disease, you know."

DR. KAHN'S OWN SPECIALTY, diabetes, is perhaps the best example of how malleable the definition of disease can be. Diabetes means "to pass through" in ancient Greek, the Greeks being the first to note the disease and its tendency, in an acute phase, to produce vast amounts of urine. Urine was likewise how the disease was diagnosed well into the 1950s, by measuring the amount of sugar, or glucose, in it. With the development of a blood glucose test, though, the conception and treatment of the disease suddenly changed. By looking for the disease in the blood, rather than in the urine, physicians could detect diabetes earlier, often before grave symptoms appeared and when it might be possible to treat the disease with insulin injections. Without treatment, diabetes is a deadly and miserable disease. With treatment, it can be endured and managed for decades.

This opportunity to get an early read on the disease also created what became known as the "iceberg theory" of diabetes: that along with the 4 million to 5 million Americans who were known to have diabetes in the 1950s, there might have been as many as 2 million more who didn't know they had either diabetes or prediabetes (along with millions in a similar ratio in other countries). The concept was revolutionary, because the definition of having true diabetes depended entirely on the blood glucose test. In 1979, that diagnostic criteria for diabetes was set at 140 milligrams of fasting glucose per deciliter of blood or higher. And in 1997 it was dropped to 126, a level that currently categorizes about 24 million Americans as having diabetes and another 60 million as having prediabetes at levels between 100 and 126 milligrams per deciliter. "Normal" levels run between 70 and 100.

But sniff at the numbers a bit and it's evident these cutoffs may create as much uncertainty as they do clarity: Does somebody who has a blood glucose level of 101 or 102 really have a disease? What's really needed for these cutoff-defined conditions is not just a way to quantify risk, but a way to calibrate it. What's needed are ways to identify risk accurately enough and early enough and strongly enough that we will be able to not only define disease early but also assess and affect the progression toward disease.

That's the idea motivating a small biotechnology company in Emeryville, California, called Tethys Bioscience, which has developed a new way to diagnose the risk for diabetes.

Medical diagnostics is, on the one hand, an industry of great innovation and invention and yet, on the other, a notoriously conservative and recalcitrant field. It is governed by the principle of a gold standard—the belief that every disease has one benchmark tool for establishing a true diagnosis. In cancer, the gold standard is a tissue biopsy; in tuberculosis, the gold standard is a culture; and in diabetes, it's the blood glucose test. The challenge for a new test, therefore, is to improve upon the gold standard in several significant ways. First and foremost, it must be equally or more accurate. Second, it should be cheaper or easier to do, or perhaps both.

A cofounder of Tethys, Mickey Urdea, PhD, and its president, Mike Richey, had spent years at Chiron, a diagnostics company, developing gold-standard tests for HIV and hepatitis C infection. They had seen many tests fail because they didn't improve upon the current standards. Along the way, though, they'd learned one lesson: One alternative to challenging the standard is to invent a new way to conceptualize a disease, to reclassify it. That's what the blood glucose test for diabetes did to the urine glucose test—it pushed the diagnosis to earlier in the disease's course and, in so doing, it changed the treatment of the condition. The idea at Tethys, then, is not to go up against the blood glucose test, but to create a test that could be used to anticipate diabetes, that could somehow predict somebody's prospects of getting diabetes.

The effort started with a list of thousands of different metabolic factors that had been associated with the various components of diabetes: obesity, metabolic syndrome, inflammation, heart disease. These components are known as biomarkers because they have properties that mark, or have been associated with, a specific condition. Scientists at Tethys were looking through the biomarkers for a handful that might closely correlate with diabetes. Then they did a bit of number crunching to find which of these biomarkers are known to exist in the blood at measurable levels *early* in the disease's course. Eventually, the company settled on seven markers. Independently, these measures didn't carry much import. But when put together in an algorithm, the markers could create what Tethys calls a Diabetes Risk Score (DRS)—a number between 1 and 10 that quantifies a person's risk of developing type 2 diabetes within 5 years.

The test, which Tethys named the PreDx Diabetes Risk Score, provides a fairly precise calculation of risk: A 7.5 equals a 10 percent risk of developing diabetes within 5 years, whereas a 9 equals a 24 percent risk. (The risk for the general population is about 3.4 percent, equal to a 5 on the PreDx scale.)

What's ingenious about PreDx is the algorithm. Unlike many new diagnostic tests trying to outdo a gold standard, the innovation isn't a technological one; it isn't quantum dots or microfluidics or nanotechnology. Instead, the smarts are in the algorithm, the number crunching. Basically, the test lets the numbers do the work, not the chemistry. Of course, the biomarker data don't themselves produce a figure on a 1-to-10 scale; they must be converted into those terms. That in and of itself is a complicated bit of biostatistics. But a patient in a doctor's office will be presented with a Diabetes Risk Score of, say, 8.1 and then shown a chart that clearly puts this at about a 13 percent risk of developing diabetes in the next 5 years. That's a lot easier for a layperson to make sense of than a blood glucose level of 113 milligrams per deciliter. Heck, it's a lot easier for a *physician* to make sense of.

Compared to a standard blood glucose test, the PreDx test isn't cheap. At $465 a pop, it's too expensive to be used as a general screening test. It's meant to be used by a physician to confirm that a patient is at an increased risk for diabetes. In other words, it's a way to pull people out of that prediabetes pool, spot their trajectory toward disease, intervene, and alter the course of a life. And it's about a *specific* life. This isn't the abstract application of population studies to an individual. This is the distillation of one person's markers, a statistically sound and personalized prediction of one person's fate.

BUT IS IT ENOUGH? Does getting a high diabetes risk score—or being diagnosed with metabolic syndrome or high blood pressure or high cholesterol or any condition that indicates a risk for another, worse condition—compel a change in behavior that actually improves health down the road?

The answer, alas, is both yes and no. Behavior change, as we saw in the last chapter, is hard. Personalized metrics, be they blood-sugar level and waist size or a PreDx score, can help people track their health. And such feedback, as we've learned, can be a powerful tool for motivating behavior change. So for many people, treating the numbers works. That's a positive sign.

But metabolic syndrome and other risk-based conditions are a specific

Scoring the Risk of Diabetes

The PreDx test, developed by Tethys Bioscience, gives individuals a score between 1 and 10 for developing diabetes over the next 5 years. A score of 8 is equal to about a 10 percent risk—but that's double the risk of an average person.

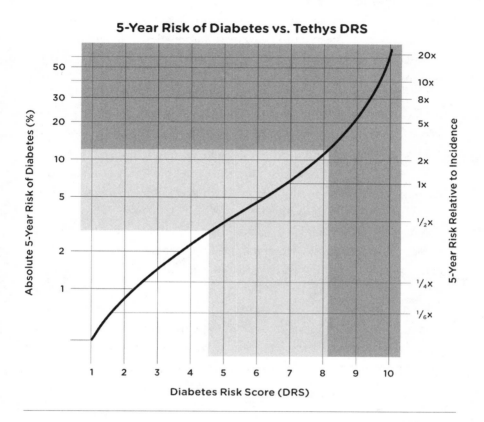

5-Year Risk of Diabetes vs. Tethys DRS

kind of feedback, one of a more pressing sort. They constitute a diagnosis, a declaration that right now, in the immediate present, *something is wrong*. This alarm—which I'll call a health crisis—can be a very effective tool for behavior change. It may wake us out of our "yeah, I'll do it someday" reverie and compel us to act.

A 2008 study of smokers and obese people in the United Kingdom found that people who experienced a health crisis were significantly more likely to change their behaviors. Some of these crises were quite harrowing: two collapsed lungs and pneumonia due to morbid obesity, chest pains in smokers, and the like. For others, the crisis was more understated: a pregnancy, or turning 30 and deciding to quit smoking once and for all. Whatever its form, a true crisis can serve as a catalyst for change, the researchers concluded, a mechanism that disrupts the course of normal life and arouses a reevaluation of identity. It puts meaning together with behavior change. A health crisis gives people permission to behave in a new way.

Such research leads naturally to the idea that a risk-based diagnosis might constitute such a crisis and therefore stir action. It sure sounds right. No doubt some people, like Carol Nelson, will consider a metabolic syndrome diagnosis to be sufficient grounds for changing their lives. But not every crisis has quite the same impact. And a risk-based diagnosis, as helpful as it can be in warding off disease, can stumble on that same rock of behavior.

As we saw in Chapter 4, compliance—getting people to adhere to recommended medical behaviors and treatments—can be tricky. Too many of us just don't do what we're told, even when it's in our best interests. An analysis of research studying patients who were prescribed medications for diabetes, high blood pressure, and high cholesterol found that only about 60 percent consistently took their medications on schedule. Patients on statins were the worst, with barely half following their prescription schedules consistently. It seems that when a diagnosis is rooted in risk for disease, rather than pegged to a symptom that causes pain or discomfort or simply makes one fret, it's less likely that pills will be taken when they should be.

If that's what happens among patients with established conditions like high cholesterol or diabetes, where does it leave a disease like metabolic syndrome? In that indefinite place, between a bona fide tool for change and a gimmick. Just as metabolic syndrome is criticized for diluting the concept of disease, so might it dilute the degree of crisis, falling short, perhaps, of the acuity needed to disrupt life enough to change it.

Engaging with our health shouldn't require us to confront our deaths, or even that we be diagnosed with a specific condition. Yes, we should know our risks. But rather than measuring them as milestones toward inevitable decline and demise, why not use them to sustain our health?

A Decision Tree approach allows us to manage our health like we do our investments. If metabolic syndrome and other risk-based diagnoses augur an era of disease portfolios, they should be secondary components in our overall health portfolios. In the long term, we should be mindful of those conditions that we are genetically predisposed for, the things we have a family history of, and take measures to fend them off. In the medium term, we should actively screen for conditions that we are perhaps trending toward so we can get a jump on intervention and treatment. And in the short term should be the day-to-day checklist of behaviors we want to engage in, as well as a list of the conditions that have already taken hold that we are actively managing.

Throughout, our overall objective should not be to avoid or manage disease. Rather, we should aim to maximize and improve our health.

Screening for Everything

When Testing Everyone for a Disease Is a Good Idea, and When It's Not

I.

IN 1963, PARENTS WERE OFFERED a new blood test for their newborns. The test screened for phenylketonuria, or PKU, a genetic disease that turns a mother's milk into poison for an affected baby. An infant with the disease can't metabolize phenylalanine, an amino acid that's present in breast milk, regular dairy products, and many other foods. A normal body processes phenylalanine without problem, and the substance is necessary for proper development. But in somebody with PKU, phenylalanine builds up in the blood and poisons the brain. Within roughly 6 months, it causes severe mental retardation. PKU occurs in about 1 of every 15,000 Americans, so it's an uncommon but not invisible disease.

The new test made it possible to detect the disease at birth. Babies with PKU could be switched to a diet low in phenylalanine, thereby avoiding the brain damage. It was considered a great triumph for public health and was one of the first newborn screening tests to be deployed across the United States.

But the test wasn't perfect. It had a significant false-positive rate; as many as 95 percent of the infants who tested positive for PKU would, with further testing, turn out *not* to have the disease. At the time, that was considered a necessary trade-off. The downside of incorrectly unnerving 95 families seemed a worthwhile side effect of finding and eliminating 5 cases of such a devastating disease. Besides, nearly all of those 95 children would be cleared upon further testing.

Nearly all—but not all. This distinction mattered, because the treatment for PKU carried side effects for children who didn't have PKU but were treated with a low-phenylalanine diet anyway. Too little phenylalanine in their diets put those normal children at an *increased* risk for mental retardation and other developmental problems. In the first few years of the test's use, as many as one in two children was being unnecessarily treated, which means the early PKU screening test could be seen as a wash. It was potentially harming just as many children as it was helping.

Over the years, the PKU test was refined and improved; today, PKU is one of a dozen diseases that newborns are routinely screened for, without incident. Indeed, newborn screening, like vaccination, is a triumph of modern medicine, quietly preventing millions of cases of disease and saving untold thousands of lives every year.

Screening tests are the prime examples of preventive medicine, the epitome of early action. Dozens of screening tests now exist for diseases ranging from Alzheimer's to stroke. The Framingham risk-score calculators for cardiovascular disease that were discussed in Chapter 1 are used to screen people, as are the prenatal genetic tests discussed in Chapter 2 and the Tethys Bioscience test for diabetes risk in Chapter 5. The hearing tests we get as schoolchildren are screening tests. Even the drug tests given to professional athletes are a form of screening. Screening tests have become a standard part of our health care. The US Preventive Services Task Force, an expert panel appointed by the Agency for Healthcare Research and Quality, recommends that a sexually active 40-year-old woman be screened regularly for a dozen conditions and lists another 19 screening tests as options. That's a lot of tests.

But the lesson of PKU is that screening tests aren't panaceas. They come with clear trade-offs for society and for individuals. False positives are the first thing to be wary of. Even when a test looks reliable—with

99 percent accuracy or higher—when it's applied to a large population to look for a rare condition, it can still result in huge numbers of false positives. Think of it this way: A test with a 99 percent accuracy rate (the test's "sensitivity," in laboratory parlance) will be wrong in only 1 test out of every 100. But if a disease occurs in only 1 of every 500 people, then 4 of every 5 positive results will be wrong, because the false positive is more common than a true case of the disease. This is how many screening tests play out. Many positives turn out to be false positives. Even for a common disease like breast cancer, which hits one in eight women in the United States, researchers estimate that about 20 percent of the women having mammograms annually will have a false-positive result during 10 years of screening.

A high false-positive rate doesn't doom a test, though. Far from it: The whole premise of screening is to cast a wide net in the hope of capturing as many cases as possible. The bycatch—the set of false positives—is simply a necessary evil. Besides, if the screening is well designed, a positive test will be followed up with a further test, ideally one that's more specific but perhaps too expensive or intricate to be widely used.

We tolerate high numbers of false positives because the alternative—false negatives—is considered even worse. A false negative means that a test has failed to identify somebody who has the disease, has given them false reassurance that they have escaped unscathed. Thus assured, these false negatives only come to light when the disease progresses into symptoms, bringing into question the whole framework and argument for the screening test. Since any test must balance false positives and false negatives, most screening tests are designed using the principle that false positives are the less egregious error and false negatives, less acceptable. The same principle applies in the law: In the United States and most democracies, the legal code is tipped toward ensuring that the wrongly accused go free, even if that means releasing some of the guilty, too. In medicine as in law, that's the balance our society has deemed best.

Besides its accuracy, though, a screening test must also be judged on its impact: Does the test actually save lives? To be more precise, are positive cases effectively treated in a way that improves lives? The question

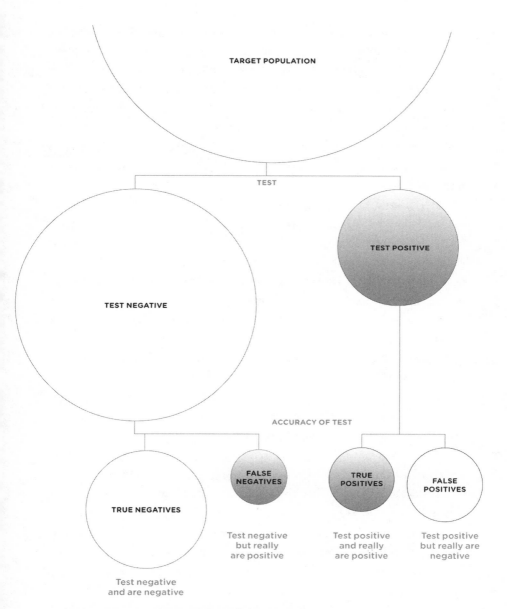

How a Screening Test Finds Disease

A screening test finds those people with disease—but typically many people who take a test get a false positive, and a small fraction get a false negative. In a good test, further testing will determine what's what.

may seem absurd—of course earlier detection means that lives are saved. But that's not always so easy to prove. Take breast cancer, for example, perhaps the most screened-for disease in the Western world. The American Cancer Society recommends annual mammogram screenings for most women ages 40 and older, and about 70 percent of American women comply. Women who receive an accurate positive result have their disease diagnosed before symptoms would have revealed the cancer. But does this early identification actually increase their survival rates? It's not so easy to tell.

Here's why. Cancer survival rates are measured from the time of diagnosis. So if a mammogram turns up a cancer 3 years earlier than it would have been discovered otherwise and the woman lives another 8 years, she'll have an 8-year postdiagnosis survival time instead of 5 years. But did that woman actually gain more years of life than she would have without mammography? It's far from clear. This is what epidemiologists call lead-time bias, and it's a huge problem in measuring the effectiveness of screening.

A good screening test, of course, accounts for all such factors. A good test minimizes the number of false positives and eliminates most false negatives. A good test is matched with a good treatment, resulting in real improvements rather than statistical anomalies. Unfortunately, not all screening tests are good tests.

There are what I'll call dumb screening and smart screening. Dumb screening is when technology is poorly used, when it proves too dazzling and obscures disease rather than clarifying it. In smart screening, the test isn't about the technology; the technology is just one part of a larger system, an algorithm that seeks to maximize the rate of true positives. Smart screening doesn't bring more experts into the equation, it lets the math do the grunt work and saves the experts until they're really needed.

IN A SCREENING TEST, THE SYSTEM IS THE KEY. A test must be applied strategically, in a framework that sorts through a large populace to identify those few individuals who, though they may show no signs, actually harbor a disease. The first step is to identify a target population that has a higher risk of a certain disease, such as those with a family history of heart disease, or men over the age of 50 who have a greater chance of developing prostate cancer, or a newborn baby who's at risk for jaundice. Where and how the cutoff is drawn has consequences. A too-narrow target population will miss some people who have the disease; a too-broad target introduces more false positives and false negatives, dilutes the hit rate, and increases costs. Since screening always results in vast numbers of negative results so a few positive cases can be rooted out, a test should be economical and, ideally, minimally invasive. A test shouldn't unnecessarily put healthy people through an ordeal only to tell them that, sure enough, nothing's wrong. A screening test should be sensitive enough to detect disease that wouldn't be discoverable through another means, such as a regular checkup. And finally, there should be an accepted and effective treatment at hand for the disease— or some measurable benefit, such as in the case of the REVEAL study's *APOE* test—to justify the effort. A well-designed screening test will navigate through this cascade of variables to hit upon unseen cases of a disease and improve lives.

In many situations, screening works. Some 30,000 children in the United States have been spared mental retardation because of PKU testing. A blood test that's used to screen for colon cancer—the second-deadliest form of cancer for men and women overall, even though, ironically, it's among the easiest to screen for—has been shown to save as many as 10,000 lives in the United States annually. These are the sorts of results that make people evangelize for screening tests. They allow the possibility of changing the future, of plucking people off one course and setting them on another toward a longer, healthier life.

And screening is only going to get more common, for three reasons. First is the emphasis on preventive medicine, based on the recognition by the medical establishment and the US government that earlier warnings save lives and money. Second is the emergence of the risk-based diseases discussed earlier: conditions like metabolic syndrome and high cholesterol that bring with them a new checklist of routine tests. The third driver is technology itself: new proxies for proximity, such as CT scans and positron-emission tomography (PET) scans, which give us a look deep inside the human body. These are tempting tools for screening large numbers of people for diseases that are otherwise invisible. Genetic tests, which skip over the imaging of our bodies and go straight to the molecular level of our cells, are another driver for more screening tests.

If these technologies are deployed systematically and wisely, they can be a great boon to our health, both collectively and individually. But the fact is that screening tests aren't always used wisely. Though a screening test can be the first step in a well-considered Decision Tree, a screening test without forethought can propel us into a zone of ambiguous probabilities and poorly calibrated risks. Screening tests demonstrate how Decision Trees sometimes are forced upon us, whether we're prepared to navigate them or not.

A screening test can set us upon a path without our understanding what we're actually testing for. We may not know the implications of a positive or negative result. A screening test can beguile us, overstating the power of technology to reveal what may or may not be going on inside our skins. But when we understand what they're good for and what they aren't, screening tests can also be opportunities. They can give us more choices. And they can fulfill their promise to improve our lives rather than fouling them up. But first, we need to understand their allure and their limitations.

II.

ANDREAS VESALIUS WAS ONLY 23 YEARS OLD when he decided to challenge 13 centuries of medical dogma. A new instructor in medicine at the University of Padua in Italy, Vesalius was intrigued by dissecting human beings—real, dead human beings. At the time—the year was 1537—this was an unusual impulse, even for a physician. Dissection carried all sorts of religious and social taboos, and, what's more, there was no need for it; the ancient Roman physician Galen had spelled out the details of human anatomy quite precisely more than 1,300 years earlier in his treatises on the human body.

But Vesalius was curious, and when he picked up his scalpel and performed his first autopsies, he was baffled by what he saw. As Vesalius looked at what lay upon his dissection table, he realized that Galen had gotten a great deal wrong. The anatomy of the heart, the flow of blood, the positions of the kidneys, the lengths of bones—it all contradicted Galen's descriptions. The father of medicine, Vesalius later said, "has departed much more than two hundred times from a true description of the harmony, use, and function of the human parts." And soon he understood why: Galen had never dissected a human. Indeed, it seemed he'd performed most of his dissections on dogs and primates.

Sixteenth-century Padua was a conservative place, and it didn't welcome Vesalius's eagerness to uproot more than a millennium of tradition. But his autopsies, which he performed in public, soon became popular affairs, drawing hundreds of university students and other spectators. When he ran short of bodies, a local judge and admirer arranged for a steady supply of the corpses of condemned criminals. Thus equipped, Vesalius began a systematic study of human anatomy. In 1543, openly challenging Galen and the status quo of European medicine, he published *De humani corporis fabrica* (*On the Fabric of the Human Body*), a seven-book masterpiece of precise anatomical drawings and penetrating erudition that stands as the first definitive document of modern medicine. Insisting that doctors begin "taking on dissections with their hands" and grapple with the messy reality of the human body, Vesalius argued that medicine was more science than art. "A knowledge of our own bodily structure is most worthy of mankind," Vesalius wrote in his introduction. All at once, he shifted his profession away from handed-down wisdom and superstition and toward empirical observation.

Vesalius's work stands as the first effort to understand what has become one of medicine's central challenges: *What's going on in there?* The last 500 years have seen a sustained effort to answer this question, an attempt to perceive the true state of human biology *before* we become corpses on the pathologist's table. The x-ray, the MRI, blood tests—these are all proxies for proximity, efforts to discern our internal biology. Cardiologists measure cholesterol levels to shed light on the state of our hearts;

radiologists beam waves of sound and light through our tissues to eke out pictures of what might be causing that pain. All of these techniques are, by necessity, approximations, full of shadows and ambiguity. Yet taken as a whole, they are remarkably good surrogates. Used as screening tests, they turn Vesalius's insistence upon empiricism and reasoning into a system, a format for peering into the body systematically even when there's no reason for it other than demographics or family history or some statistical justification. They suggest that Vesalius's question can be answered, that the state of the human body can be perceived, at least approximately, when it still matters: when we're still alive.

IF YOU'RE LOOKING FOR A SCAPEGOAT for the escalating cost of health care—$2 trillion a year in the United States, and climbing—you might as well blame the Beatles.

In 1931, Electric and Musical Industries, or EMI, was mostly about the *M*—making 78 rpm records and selling gramophones. The *E* was a much smaller part of the company, one in which EMI engineers worked on military technologies and dabbled in the burgeoning field of computer electronics (EMI labs helped develop radar technology and stereo sound, among other things). In 1955, the company acquired Capitol Records, with its roster of Frank Sinatra, Nat "King" Cole, and Peggy Lee, and became a powerhouse in popular music.

And in 1962, on the recommendation of EMI recording executive George Martin, the company signed a new group called the Beatles to a recording contract. Over the next decade (and for years thereafter) the company earned millions of dollars from the Fab Four. It was so much money that the company almost didn't know what to do with it.

Meanwhile, a middle-aged bachelor engineer named Godfrey Hounsfield was working at EMI's less glamorous electronics business. Hounsfield was a skilled but unassuming scientist, quietly leading a team that built the first all-transistor computer. Hounsfield's success with computers had earned him goodwill on the science side of the company and, flush with money broken out of teenagers' piggy banks, EMI let Hounsfield pursue independent research.

One day in 1967—the year of *Sgt. Pepper's Lonely Hearts Club Band* and *Magical Mystery Tour*—Hounsfield took a ramble through the English countryside and had an epiphany. By taking a picture of an object from all sides, he realized, one could create a three-dimensional image of that object. He went back to his lab and was soon taking x-rays of a cow's head (borrowed from a nearby slaughterhouse) from all sides. By converting the images into digital files, rather than strips of film, Hounsfield discovered that a computer could reassemble dozens or hundreds of x-rays into one single image, creating a deeper look inside the head. The result was a cross-sectional, interior image with remarkable clarity. He called the technique computed tomography, or CT. As the Nobel Prize committee put it in awarding Hounsfield the Nobel Prize in Physiology or Medicine in 1979, before the CT scanner, "ordinary X-ray examinations of the head had shown the skull bones, but the brain had remained a gray, undifferentiated fog. Now, suddenly, the fog had cleared."

First released as a clinical scanner by EMI in 1971 (the year after the Beatles broke up), CT scanners started to appear at hospitals in the mid-1970s. Today, there are about 30,000 in use worldwide, one-third of them in the United States.

CT technology has been a boon to medicine, aiding in the diagnosis of everything from broken bones to kidney disease to cancer. CT images of the brain—the use that Hounsfield designed them for—brought clarity that would have dumbfounded Vesalius.

But as we'll see, CT scans have also been a major factor in the explosion of health care costs in the United States. These days, these very expensive machines—along with their high-resolution brethren, MRIs and PET scans—are sometimes used indiscriminately, often in an effort to generate a diagnosis rather than confirm one. Despite their high resolution, CT scans are still blunt instruments. They can actually introduce *too much* information into a situation. A high-resolution image of the inside of the body reveals so much that everything begins to look like an anomaly or a potential problem. As Shannon Brownlee wrote in her 2007 book *Overtreated*, "for every scan that helps a physician come to the right decision, another scan may cloud the picture, sending the doctor down the wrong path."

Despite these limitations, CT scans are not only being used to diagnose disease. They're also being recommended for screening purposes for heart disease, cancer, and other chronic diseases. And that makes them a prime example of dumb screening.

MOST TECHNOLOGIES GET CHEAPER as they get more popular. DVD players, digital cameras, flat-screen televisions, and pretty much every other technology you can think of has undergone this: The more people who buy them, and the more the technology improves, the cheaper the product gets. This is the wonder of Moore's law, the steady and exponential improvement of computer circuitry, processing, and memory that makes all things digital cheaper and better. But that's not at all what's happened with CT scans.

The resolution of a CT scan is measured in slices. Each rotation of the x-ray unit around an object generates a certain number of cross-sectional images; those cross-sections are called slices. The more slices per rotation, the higher the resolution of the image, just like a higher-resolution digital camera produces a sharper image. Since the 1990s, CT scans have leapt from 4 to 8 to 16 to 32 to 64 slices, with a dramatic improvement in the quality of the machines. Yet the price of CT scanners has stayed consistently and breathtakingly high. From 1974 to 2004, the list price of a CT scanner increased from $385,000 to $2.2 million, a nearly sixfold increase (with inflation accounting for only about $1 million of that increase). Sure, that $2.2 million buys a better machine than $385,000 did 30 years ago. But the price arrow points in the opposite direction from that seen with other technologies, where the economics of scale and Moore's law have consistently driven costs down, even as quality goes up.

So what's going on with CT machines? It's a paradox that's worth understanding better, because the explanation hints at why health care costs in general keep going up—and why technology-intensive screening may not be such a smart idea.

Economists have a term for industries that don't follow conventional economic rules of competition and efficiency: market failures. The health

How Technology Raises Health Care Costs

In contrast to consumer technologies like computers, which get cheaper every year, in health care, technologies, like CT scanners, get more expensive.

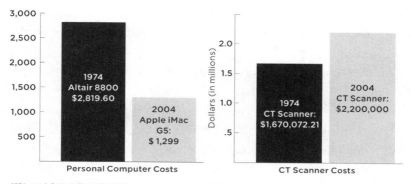

1974 costs inflation adjusted for 2004
SOURCES: Radiology Management, Computer History Museum, Apple, US Office of Technology Assessment

care industry is beset by market failure. One reason is price transparency. In a competitive market, buyers of a service can glean what a typical price for a service or commodity is, and sellers will know what their competitors are selling their products for. This creates a fair market where buyers can shop around and sellers can adjust their prices to maximize either sales or profit. The marketplace for CT scanners, alas, has very little transparency. The same manufacturer may sell the same type of machine at drastically different prices to different hospitals in the same city, depending on previous contracts and relationships.

This opacity hasn't kept hospitals from buying the machines in great numbers. Following their own perverse economics, hospitals and other medical providers—including doctor's offices—have spent the past decade eagerly buying ever more powerful and ever more expensive devices. Despite a general prohibition against ordering tests simply because there's a test to order—what's called physician-induced care—that's exactly what happens. Having made their investment, hospitals put the machines to use, and a spending cycle kicks in. Doctors in the United States ordered nearly 70 million CT scans in 2007, more than triple the number in 1995. These numbers will only keep going up: As demand for imaging rises, incentive to buy new machines rises, too. Sales of imaging equipment in the United States are expected to grow from $7.8 billion in 2007 to $11.6 billion by 2012. That's why radiology departments have become profit centers for hospitals, and that's why imaging machines are exhibit A in the rising cost of health care in the United States.

This points to a second cause of market failure: Hospitals pass along the expense of CT scans to both patients and insurers. That passing along means they don't experience a downside to their actions (creating what economists call a moral hazard). And without a downside, they just keep ordering more tests: Medicare alone saw its payments to physicians for imaging services double to about $14 billion from 2000 to 2006, according to a US Government Accountability Office report issued in June 2008.

And there's a third factor at work, too: In most industries, technology lowers costs by reducing the workload for an expert class. The steam engine reduced the demand for buggy whip makers, the textile factory reduced the need for seamstresses, robot welders reduced the need for the human kind in auto plants. But here again, health care is the exception: Rather than taking experts out of the process, a CT scan ends up making *more* work for the expert class of radiologists. Diagnostic radiology is routinely among the highest-paid specialties in medicine, with a median salary of $463,000, according to a 2008 survey of specialties. And these salaries are increasing faster than they are for other MDs, driven by hospitals that are eager for more radiologists to perform more tests. That not only keeps prices high, it makes the prospects for lowering costs almost nonexistent.

Clayton Christensen, DBA, a professor at Harvard Business School and author of *The Innovator's Prescription,* has cited this as one of the reasons health care is in such dire straits. "When you deploy the technology to commoditize the caregiver, to enable a lower-cost provider to do something that historically had required higher cost, then it actually takes cost out of the system," he told the policy journal *Health Affairs* in 2007. But, he said, "when you bring technology to the experts to do more sophisticated things, in fact, it does bring a lot of cost into the system." The result is a classic perversion of technology and economics.

All of this would argue that CT scanners are particularly ill suited as a tool for screening. After all, they fail to meet several standards of a good test. They offer no economies of scale; the machines don't get cheaper when you buy more, and the individual scans don't get cheaper when you scan more people. And they don't give unequivocal information; unlike a blood test quantifying blood glucose level, a scan is open to a radiologist's interpretation. It's for these reasons that the US Preventive Services Task Force has consistently recommended against using CT scans to screen for diseases. CT scans also carry some risk of radiation exposure, a risk that increases with the frequency of the scans.

But those objections haven't stopped the tide. Other groups, such as the American College of Cardiology and the American Cancer Society, insist that CT scans are worthwhile for screening for coronary heart disease, lung and colon cancers, and even any number of blips or blobs that whole-body scans may turn up. Such uses, as I'll explain, are deeply controversial, especially when they venture beyond high-risk groups into a more general population. It's as if the look that Vesalius first gave us deep inside the human body has proven hypnotic.

A CT SCAN OF THE LUNGS is a beautiful thing to behold. Compared with the foggy blur of an x-ray, the lungs are revealed in sharp, exquisite detail. The lobes show up as networks of rivers, with the bronchioles that conduct air from the trachea fanning out into the alveoli, one tributary branching into a hundred more. Any unusual blip, be it from infection or cancer, shows up on this map as a well-defined land mass with a precise longitude and latitude.

In the mid-1990s, the International Early Lung Cancer Action Program (I-ELCAP) began a 12-year study to examine the potential of CT scans as a screening tool for the disease. The study brought 30,000 smokers into hospitals and scanned their lungs, following up with another scan a year or so later. The scans turned up 484 cases of potential cancer, and subsequent biopsies confirmed that 85 percent of those patients did indeed have stage I lung cancer. It was a stunning result, far higher than many would have predicted. Even more remarkable was the survival rate: Of the 375 patients who opted for surgery, 92 percent were still alive 10 years later. The triumphant findings, published in 2006 in the *New England Journal of Medicine,* seemed to make a clear case for the widespread use of CT scans as a screening test for the early detection of lung cancer. "I consider it reasonable for older smokers and others at high risk of lung cancer to talk to their physician about having annual CT screening," Claudia Henschke, MD, PhD, a physician at the New York-Presbyterian Hospital/Weill Cornell Medical College and lead author of the *NEJM* study, said at the time.

But there's one question the study didn't ask: "What if they're finding things that look like cancer—even things that may be cancer under the microscope—but that aren't the cancers that actually kill people?" asks Peter Bach, MD, a pulmonologist at Memorial Sloan-Kettering Cancer Center in New York. Dr. Bach's concern was that, by itself, a CT scan makes it too easy to rush to judgment.

Dr. Bach had strong enough doubts about the conclusion drawn from I-ELCAP that he decided to do his own assessment of CT screening for lung cancer. He collected the results from three other large studies of CT scans among smokers in the United States and Italy. As I-ELCAP had, these studies found that, yes, CT scans detected a huge number of early cancers—10 times more than they would expect to find without scanning. In that regard, the scans seemed to do their job as a screening test. And as expected, the number of surgeries based on those diagnoses jumped. But when Dr. Bach looked at the resulting mortality rates, he found essentially no difference between those who had received a CT scan and those who had not. Despite the additional surgeries, just as many people were dying as before. And in this regard, CT scans seemed to be a failure as a screening test—they didn't appear to save any lives at all.

So if these aren't all lethal cancers, what are the CT scans finding? Dr. Bach believes it's what some radiologists call pseudodisease. His theory is that lung cancer may come in at least two forms: fast-growing, lethal tumors that appear "like a meteor" and spread quickly, and slow-growing masses that are essentially benign. This isn't the same thing as an imprecise test turning up false positives or false negatives—on a molecular level, these are real cancers. They're just not the kinds of tumors that would eventually kill a patient.

And if CT scans are finding primarily the slow-growing types, then the test may be doing more harm than good when you consider the trauma lung surgery entails. The procedure requires cutting through layers of muscle, nerves, and, depending on the position of the tumor, sometimes bone before a lobe of the lung is removed. As many as 2 percent to 5 percent of patients die from the procedure. Recovery is slow and painful, and lifelong consequences include an increased risk of cardiovascular problems. "If you have to whack out a large part of their lung, we should be much more careful," says Dr. Bach.

As for Dr. Henschke, her research came under a different sort of scrutiny after it was revealed that funding for the I-ELCAP study could be traced back to a $3.6 million grant from the Vector Group, a parent company of the Liggett Group, a major tobacco company that produces several brands of cigarettes. Why would a tobacco company want to fund research into lung cancer? Perhaps because if lung cancer can be cured, smoking may not seem so bad.

And then there was the matter of the 27 patent applications submitted by Dr. Henschke and her colleagues related to lung cancer screening. It turned out that they had a licensing agreement with General Electric, a major manufacturer of CT scanners, for a computer algorithm they developed to detect lung cancer on diagnostic images. The more often CT scans were used to screen for lung cancer, the more Dr. Henschke and her partners would make. The GE deal wasn't disclosed in any of her papers.

The lesson of the lung cancer screening debacle is that technology isn't a panacea. It must be used wisely, systematically, and after directing a cold eye toward determining whether the rewards outweigh the risks. Such measures are the standard to which all screening should be subjected. They are the hallmarks of the most successful screening test, in terms of lives saved, that medicine has yet come up with: the Pap test.

III.

IN 1923, GEORGE PAPANICOLAOU had a eureka moment. A Greek-born pathologist working at Cornell Medical College in New York City, Dr. Papanicolaou was in his lab inspecting some tissues that had been scraped off women's cervixes. As he peered through his microscope, he saw some unusual cells come into focus. He realized that they were cancer cells and, what's more, that he could clearly identify them as such, based only on a simple swipe of the cervix.

"The first observation of cancer cells in the smear of the uterine cervix gave me one of the greatest thrills I ever experienced during my scientific career," he later wrote. In 1928, after spending a few years refining his research, Dr. Papanicolaou eagerly presented his technique at a Michigan medical conference. Though he had anticipated great acclaim, his findings were ignored. The conventional method for diagnosing cervical cancer—a full biopsy—was considered the only definitive test for cancer. It was the gold standard. Anything else was waved off as useless speculation.

But Dr. Papanicolaou realized that a biopsy was often done too late for many women, and he persisted in his work. In 1943 he published a paper entitled "Diagnosis of Uterine Cancer by the Vaginal Smear," providing the first definitive evidence that a Pap test could effectively detect not just a cervical cancer but also a lesion that was very likely to turn into cancer soon enough.

Though it would still be another 20 years before the Pap test was a standard part of women's health care, Dr. Papanicolaou had at last prevailed. His test worked, and it has proven to be the most effective preventive measure ever devised against any cancer. Every American woman is now advised to have a routine Pap test at least every 3 years once she becomes sexually active. Rates of cervical cancer have fallen by 50 to 70 percent in most developed nations (by three-quarters in the

United States)—a statistic all the more remarkable because so many other cancers have proven so resistant to early detection.

The Pap test has become the template for an effective screening test: a simple, mildly intrusive test that requires little advanced technology but can detect a disease years before it would otherwise become evident. Millions of women are alive today because of it.

THE PAP TEST ISN'T PERFECT. For one thing, the test has a very high false-negative rate—it may miss as many as 45 percent of cases, according to Eduardo Franco, DrPH, an epidemiologist and expert in cervical cancer screening at McGill University in Montreal. This high false-negative rate means that women should get the test fairly often so a cancer missed in one year can be spotted the next. But that frequency creates its own danger, since the more tests that are required, the more likely it is that a woman will skip one. "Even here in Canada, where we have free tests and free health care—so you'd think it'd be unthinkable to have someone come down with the disease—some people do get cancer," says Dr. Franco. "The test process is flawed."

These limitations have led Dr. Franco and others to search for an alternative to the Pap test, one that is equally easy—or easier—to use but catches more true positive cases of the disease. And they may have found it. In early 2009, a team from the International Agency for Research on Cancer published a study in the *New England Journal of Medicine* that screened more than 130,000 women in India for human papillomavirus (HPV), the virus believed to cause nearly all cases of cervical cancer. Like a Pap test, the HPV test starts with scraping the cervix. But whereas a Pap test is sent to a laboratory for analysis, which typically takes a few days, the HPV sample is inserted into a machine that analyzes the tissue for the virus's genetic signal. In a couple of hours, the machine can determine whether HPV DNA is present.

This machine-driven process effectively automates a procedure that otherwise requires significant expertise. It allows technology to do the job more efficiently, precisely as Dr. Christensen and others advocate. The implications are huge. Automation means the test can be done more cheaply—for as little as $5 a test, rather than $50 or so for a Pap test—and can be used much more widely. The study, for instance, was conducted in India, rather than in the United States or Europe, to demonstrate that it would work in a country without a robust laboratory infrastructure.

What's more, testing for the presence of HPV DNA, rather than for early stage cancer cells, means the test isn't detecting disease, but rather singling out women with an *increased risk* of disease developing over the next few years. Identifying these women earlier means they can first be singled out and *then* followed with a Pap test to catch disease much earlier. Dr. Franco calls this the "algorithm for treatment"—using a series of tests to statistically sort a large population with a low risk of disease into a smaller population with a higher risk. "By being upstream in the natural history of the disease, there's an even better chance to save lives," says Dr. Franco enthusiastically. "There's a better window of opportunity."

Women who test negative for HPV, meanwhile, can be spared frequent testing, because the false-negative problem with Pap tests no longer applies. They only need to return every 3 years or so for another DNA test. "The beauty is that when it's negative, the DNA test provides much more assurance to the woman," Dr. Franco adds. "On a Pap [test], there was always this doubt about a negative test, and they'd have at most 1 year of assurance. But now you get 3 or 4 years of peace of mind. The algorithm is a much more winning combination."

But the success of cervical cancer screening is the exception among screening tests, not the rule. For one thing, the Pap test wouldn't have happened if not for the decades-long persistence of Dr. Papanicolaou. He researched and developed and advocated his discovery in the face of great resistance from those who supported the status quo (many feel that he was cruelly denied a Nobel Prize for his work, which has saved far more lives than the work of many of the scientists who received the prize during his lifetime). This against-the-odds scenario repeated itself in the effort to develop an HPV test. The India study and the development of a

$5 test didn't just happen. They were financed by the Bill and Melinda Gates Foundation, a group with exceptional resources. The test wasn't the fruit of typical scientific research, or of typical market forces (few diagnostic companies, for instance, would bother to spend a decade developing a test worth just $5 a pop).

And the new DNA test is exceptional in another way, too: It uses technology in the right way. Rather than creating a complicated process that brings more experts into the process, the HPV test actually *removes* humans from the equation. Indeed, it lets the algorithm be the equation (so to speak). It keeps the experts on retainer, as it were, until a point in the diagnostic process when their judgment is indispensable. It is screening done smartly.

IV.

IF THIS CHAPTER WERE ABOUT TESTING BRIDGES or buildings instead of bodies, there would be one more consideration before any test was deemed smart or effective: Do the benefits outweigh the costs?

Cost-benefit analysis is a concept that's been around since 1849, when the French engineer Jules Dupuit assessed the trade-offs in whether people would be willing to pay a bridge toll. The principle is straightforward: Any positive benefits (getting to the other side of the bridge) are weighed against all the negatives (the cost of the toll, the time it takes to make the crossing) before a decision to act is made. For assessing the value of government and industry projects, cost-benefit analysis has been standard practice since the 1930s.

Medicine, alas, has come late to this particular party. For decades, the prevailing wisdom in health care has been to spare no expense, to throw every tool and test and scan and procedure at a patient at the discretion of the doctor and (to a lesser extent) the insurer. This principle has lowered the bar for ordering a screening test. The *system* of screening—the winnowing of the potential population for screening that limits

A Decision Tree for Cervical Cancer Screening

The advent of a new DNA test for human papillomavirus, the principle cause of cervical cancer, means that women can be tested earlier and less frequently than with the Pap test alone. But the HPV DNA test is just the first of several circumstances that must be considered.

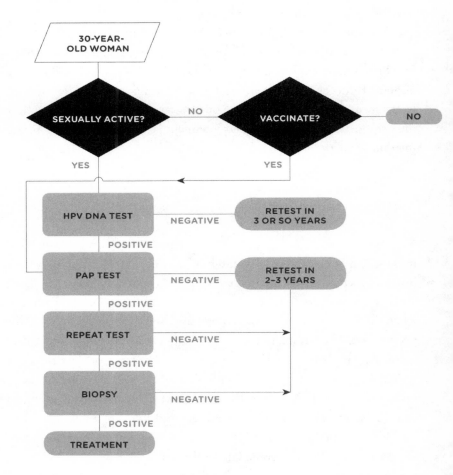

it to the most likely candidates—is often neglected, leading to the wrong tests being given to the wrong people. The results are increased costs, needless worrying, and even unnecessary treatments.

Prior to the mid-1970s, the costs, benefits, and consequences of screening tests weren't subjected to too much thought. A test was a test, and a treatment was a treatment, and they weren't really considered to be two sides of the same coin. It wasn't until 1975, when Jerome Kassirer, MD, and Stephen Pauker, MD, published a paper in the *New England Journal of Medicine,* that the idea of cost-benefit analysis truly came to medicine. Dr. Kassirer and Dr. Pauker suggested that physicians should weigh a treatment against the likelihood that a patient actually has a condition; the more reliable the test, the lower the "therapeutic threshold" for administering a treatment. "If the probability of disease in a given patient exceeds the threshold, the preferable course of action is to treat," they wrote. "If the probability is below the threshold, the preferable course of action is to withhold treatment."

Take the example of skin cancer. The screening test for melanoma, as recommended by the American Academy of Dermatology and the American Cancer Society, couldn't be more low tech (albeit expert dependent): If you are over a certain age, a dermatologist should occasionally do a full-body inspection of your skin, from head to toe. Anything that looks suspicious is removed in a quick surgical procedure. Because it's relatively easy to find and easy to treat, survival rates for melanoma are among the highest for any cancer. The argument for screening, therefore, is straightforward: Even though it requires an expensive expert, the treatment is easy and effective enough to justify broad screening. It falls above the threshold.

Lung cancer, as I explained above, is pretty much the opposite. Treatment is exceptionally difficult and dangerous and can have fatal consequences in and of itself. A diagnosis needs to be particularly definitive in such cases, and the argument for broad screening, therefore, is harder to justify.

Dr. Kassirer went on to take the top job at *NEJM,* acting as editor-in-chief of what is still among the most influential publications in medicine. For nearly a decade, he advanced the cause of smart screening, publishing studies that exposed the risks as well as the rewards of driving people toward medical treatment. Moreover, he advocated that patients should always be fully informed about tests and empowered to make their own decisions. "Even if screening confers a small benefit, a woman might choose not to be tested," he wrote in an editorial about mammography screening in 1997. "As physicians, our job is to analyze the data, assess our patients' risks as best we can, and then inform, explain, and advise."

Though such advice may seem commonsensical, Dr. Kassirer's notion of weighing the costs of screening as well as the benefits (and including patients in the decision making) still is often neglected. Talk to him today—30 years after he first suggested the idea of pinpointing a threshold for treatment—and his voice rises in frustration. "The point was, suppose you have a disease in which the treatment is very risky—say, chemotherapy for cancer. In that situation, you must be certain you have the disease before you treat. On the other hand, if you have a disease that's very low risk for treatment, then you can treat. We put chlorine in the water: We treat everyone for salmonella, because the risk is negligible.

"There is an enormous enthusiasm for preventing disease by using screening," Dr. Kassirer continues. "But enthusiasm is not enough. There's insufficient attention being paid to cost and to false positives and false negatives and to the consequences."

Consequences is exactly the word, because too often in screening, plenty of attention is paid to the quality and interpretation of the results (whether a positive is a true positive, for example), but scant mind is paid to what is to be *done* with the results. When a screening test yields a positive, are the consequences for the patient clear? Have they been thought out in advance? Is there a game plan for what a patient should do *following* the test? Often enough, there's been little or no discussion of these consequences. But there are some efforts to change that, to provide people undergoing a screening procedure with a picture of what lies on the other side of the test. And sometimes, patients are creating these tools themselves.

WHEN TOM NEVILLE WAS TOLD he had prostate cancer at age 54, he thought he knew exactly what the costs and benefits were: Unless he got treatment, he was going to die. As he saw it, he had two choices. He could undergo radiation therapy and hope to kill the cancer but save his prostate. Or he could have his prostate removed, which would be nearly certain to eliminate the cancer but carried significant risks of incontinence and impotence.

What Neville didn't realize at the time, though, is that his case was at best a toss-up and perhaps didn't meet the threshold for treatment at all. Though prostate cancer sounds horrible, the truth is that more than half of men have some cancer in their prostates by age 80, but less than 5 percent of those diagnosed actually die of the disease. These odds mean that, statistically speaking, the vast majority of men who have prostate cancer don't need treatment. In fact, as Neville says now, most men shouldn't even get a biopsy. What they don't know, he argues, probably won't hurt them. The problem is that the mainstream approach to prostate cancer points in the direction of biopsy and treatment without pausing to consider the treatment threshold.

The confusion starts with the screening test for prostate cancer itself—the PSA test. Short for prostate-specific antigen, PSA is a protein produced by the prostate gland. The PSA test measures the level of PSA in the blood. Some amount (around 1 nanogram per milliliter or more) is common, but a level of 4 or higher is considered suspicious of cancer (though some suggest that the suspicion threshold should be lowered to 3). As the number creeps over 4, the reasoning goes, the probability rises that there is cancer. Of course, the test doesn't actually measure cancer; it measures the amount of PSA, and there are all sorts of causes for a high PSA level besides cancer, starting with inflammation or infection. Still, a high PSA typically leads to a biopsy, and since so many older men have some trace of detectable cancer, it's not unusual to find something. But remember—just because there's cancer doesn't mean it's a lethal cancer. In other words, a high PSA level could prompt discovery of a coincidence, revealing a cancer that's probably never going to be a problem.

Tom Neville never properly understood this when he was considering treatment. Instead, when he got his diagnosis, he says, "I spent hours in the library. I was going cross-eyed reading research articles, trying to make sense of all this." What he did know was that his biopsy results had scared him. And no matter what the statistics were, "I had this emotional fear. I had a visceral reaction, to not want a cancer growing inside me. It was a get-it-out-of-me syndrome." And so on April 25, 2002, he had his prostate removed.

Even after his surgery, though, Neville, an engineer by training, kept poring over the research. Eventually he realized that he may not have needed surgery at all, given his low risk of dying from prostate cancer. But that information would have come in handy *before* his biopsy, before the word *cancer* had come into play with all its emotional associations. And he realized that it should be possible to give men more information sooner, so that they can assess their options before they get scared to death about a cancer inside them. Maybe the PSA test could start a process rather than compel a treatment. Maybe it would be possible to give people more choices, sooner.

What he came up with is Soar BioDynamics, a company that sells a decision-support tool for men who are trying to make sense of their PSA test results. The idea is to discern what, exactly, besides cancer could produce a high PSA level, so men don't move too quickly toward biopsy and removal, with all the latter's negative consequences. Using the information from a man's PSA test along with that from a few other easy tests and data points, Neville's tool calculates the most likely scenarios for what's happening inside a man's body, ranging from an enlarged prostate, to an infection, to a lethal cancer. The calculations are presented as probability scores for diagnoses. "We can cut way down on the false positives and eliminate detection of the cancers that aren't progressing. You want to catch the bad stuff but ignore the stuff you don't need to know about," he says. "Instead of a biopsy and surgery, maybe you just need to take an aspirin to cut down on the inflammation, or take antibiotics to take care of an infection."

Neville, who considers himself an acolyte of Clayton Christensen, is especially proud of how the Soar system has automated expertise. The computer model is based on published research, the same papers that made Neville scratch his head in the library back in 2002. But in this case, it customizes the research, flipping it from an abstraction into something tailored to an individual's circumstances. It turns this great heap of science into a basis for making clearer decisions.

"The issue isn't just what decisions you make, but what order you make them in," says Neville. "We're trying to switch the order of events. There's all this stuff driving people toward biopsy and treatment. We'd like to eliminate the unnecessary biopsies and only go to the expensive experts when it's highly warranted. We're not trying to do away with screening. The PSA test can be a valuable test; there's a lot of information in there. But it's important to know what the test actually shows."

Soar charges for its service—$80 for 1 year of reports. But there are other, free tools out there that take a similar approach, turning research around so an individual can interrogate it for its applicability to his specific circumstances, rather than having to navigate through stacks of research papers and findings for some wisp of relevance.

The University of Texas at San Antonio, for instance, has developed a prostate risk calculator that lets a man enter his PSA level along with his age, race, family history, and a couple of other metrics and churns out his risk of developing prostate cancer. Importantly, the calculator also calculates the risk of a *high-grade* cancer, accounting for the fact that not all prostate cancers are lethal. The value of such a tool, says Ian M. Thompson, MD, professor and chairman of the department of urology at the University of Texas Health Science Center at San Antonio, who developed the calculator, is that it turns the PSA figure from one isolated data point into one of many inputs. "We need to build in characteristics about the person, their age, their race, their family history," says Dr. Thompson. "It's not just what one test tells us."

The technical term for a calculator like this is a nomogram, a predictive tool that combines information on one patient with a body of previously established data from large populations (a body mass index, or BMI, calculator, in which you simply enter your weight and height to get your BMI, is a very simple kind of nomogram). Nomograms are one of the best examples of Decision Tree medicine, the sorts of tools that are easy for patients and doctors alike to use and understand—particularly when they're available online and free of charge. The Framingham risk calculators are a kind of nomogram. Memorial Sloan-Kettering Cancer Center, the research institute and hospital in New York City, has developed almost a dozen nomograms for a range of medical conditions. There are tools for predicting the spread of breast cancer, a tool for assessing lung cancer risk among smokers, a tool for predicting the prognosis after colon cancer surgery, and more.

Nomograms are especially powerful when they're combined with a screening test, because they help people understand what to make of the test and point to what to do with the result. They immediately customize the clinical data, be they nanograms-per-milliliter figures or spots on mammograms. Nomograms let patients ignore the inscrutable repository of jargon that is medical research in favor of something personal, something real, and something to go on. They allow us to make sense of a screening test's result, and allow us to take some measure of meaning from it.

FIVE HUNDRED YEARS after Vesalius first offered us the techniques for devising sound medicine, it's high time for us to stop being dazzled by the ability to look inside the body and start applying hard, cold rigor to the task. The ability to see inside the body is an awesome thing, but we should no longer be awestruck by it. Rather, we should use technology for what it's best suited for—removing humans from the initial process of screening, leaving human expertise for more subjective considerations.

Thankfully, the distinction between smart screening and dumb screening seems to be making inroads. Drawing on research by Dr. Thompson and others, in late 2009 the American Cancer Society, which had long advocated screening at all costs, acknowledged that for some cancers screening can do more harm than good. "We don't want people to panic," Otis Brawley, MD, chief medical officer of the Cancer Society, told the *New York Times*. "But I'm admitting that American medicine has overpromised when it comes to screening. The advantages to screening have been exaggerated." It was a significant shift, because it acknowledged that our approach to screening must contend with the complexity of disease.

In the next chapter, I'll take a close look at one effort to devise a smart screening test for cancer from scratch. If it works, it could be a template for other tests to detect cancers years before we now find them.

7

Canaries in the Coal Mine

Why Detecting Disease Is More Complicated
Than We Had Hoped It Would Be

I.

WHEN THE FIRST CELL in Brenda Rosenthal's ovary mutated and turned cancerous, she had no symptoms. The telltale pains or lumps that signal cancer were still months, if not years, away. But there were signs, sparks thrown off by the tumor that had begun to flame in her belly. As each cell was detoured from its original task, the one coded in its DNA, and conscripted for a new, malignant goal, it seeped proteins into Brenda's bloodstream. But there was no way to detect these signs, so they went unheeded.

Certainly, there were statistical flags, if Brenda, a Brooklyn native now living in Delray Beach, Florida, had known to look for them. She had survived a bout with breast cancer 20 years before, increasing her risk of developing ovarian cancer down the line. But Brenda never thought to get tested. "It didn't even register. I went on with my life, and I didn't think about cancer. I guess I was noncompliant," she says, using the term for a patient who fails to follow up on her treatment (in other words, a person who forgets she's a patient). So it wasn't until she was presented with a physical symptom in 2005—"this huge lump in my stomach area"—that Brenda learned that she was no longer a cancer survivor, but once again a cancer patient.

Ovarian cancer, like most other cancers, is measured in four stages. Stage I is early, when the disease is contained in the ovaries. In stage II, it may also be present in the fallopian tubes or elsewhere in the pelvis. By stage III, it has migrated further into the abdomen or to the lymph nodes. And by stage IV, the malignancy has spread, or metastasized, to the insides of major organs like the liver and lungs. (The first three stages are further subdivided into A, B, and C levels.) For ovarian tumors discovered in stage I or II, the survival rate 10 years after diagnosis is reassuringly high—almost 90 percent—because treatment is straightforward: surgery, perhaps followed by low doses of radiation. But survival rates drop precipitously as the diagnosis shifts to stage III or IV, when the cancer is well established and spreading. Here, the survival rate falls to 60 percent and then to 20 percent. Unfortunately, more than two-thirds of ovarian cancers aren't found until these later stages. That was true in Brenda Rosenthal's case: By the time she noticed her lump, the disease had spread and progressed to stage IIIC.

Four years later, after two rounds of chemotherapy, Brenda's cancer is in remission. But she remains vigilant. Every 3 months, her blood is tested for its level of CA-125, a protein marker used to monitor ovarian cancer. She tracks clinical drug trials in the hope that she will qualify as a subject. Yet she'll always blame herself, if only a little bit, for not finding the disease earlier. "I could live 10 or 15 years more, but I still won't have the quality of life I would've if we'd found the cancer early," she says. "I don't want anyone else to be in my position."

THE TROUBLE WITH CANCER is that it gives us too many stories like Brenda's. We want medicine to spare no effort in curing her, and we want her to defy the odds and survive. And it's right to do so. But the stories don't only distort the way we talk about cancer—as a war, a race to a cure, a test of character—they also distort the way we see the disease. They distort our perspective, and they distort our science.

The survival rates for many cancers resemble the cliff that characterizes survival of ovarian malignancies. Find the disease in stage I or II, thanks to a stray blob on an x-ray or an early symptom, and the odds of survival approach 90 percent. The treatment is surgery, and it is typically low risk. But find it late, after the tumor has metastasized, and the treatment turns violent, with infusions of toxic chemicals and blasts of brutal radiation. And here the prognosis is as miserable as the experience.

This reality would seem to make a plain case for shifting the research priority and resources toward the patients with a 90 percent, rather than a 10 or 20 percent, chance of survival. But these are largely hypothetical patients, because only one-third of ovarian cancers are found in stages I and II. The much larger number of women diagnosed when their ovarian cancers are at stage III or IV, however, are very real. They are our mothers, our daughters, and our friends. They're right in front of us. They are among the 560,000 Americans who die of cancer every year. So it's hard to shift the research and resources away from treating these difficult cases.

Billions of dollars have been spent in developing treatments that might—maybe—save these late-stage patients with better drugs that try to kill a cancer when it is at its strongest. This cure-what's-already-gone-wrong approach has dominated cancer research since President Richard Nixon declared war on the disease in 1971. But it has yielded meager results: The overall cancer mortality rate in the United States fell by a scant 9 percent from 1975 to 2006, and much of that is attributable to behavior change, such as quitting smoking, rather than some magic medicine. (Heart disease deaths, by comparison, dropped by nearly 60 percent.) We are so consumed by the quest to save the 560,000 that we overlook the far more staggering statistic on the other side of the survival curve: More than a third of all Americans—some 120 million people—will be diagnosed with cancer sometime in their lives. Some of them are out there now, though their illnesses may remain invisible until they're more advanced. And that presents a great and largely unexamined opportunity: Find and treat their cancers early, and that 560,000 figure will drop.

Cancer, you might say, has a perception problem. We have a limited ability to see what's going on inside the body on a minute scale, to gaze through the too-solid flesh and glean information on a molecular level. That's the promise of a screening test for cancer—or, more accurately,

The Riddle of Early Detection

More than 120 million Americans will get cancer at some point in their lives. Find the disease early, and survival rates are high. Catch it late, and it's much more likely to be fatal. There are three main hurdles to clear before widespread early detection becomes possible (see below).

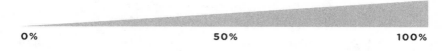

| 0% | 50% | 100% |

CUMULATIVE PERCENTAGE OF PEOPLE DIAGNOSED AT EACH STAGE

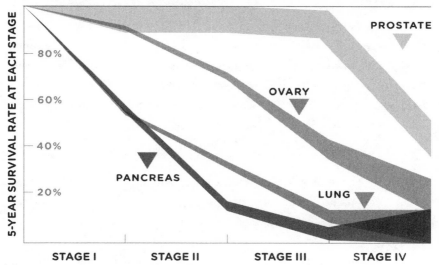

5-YEAR SURVIVAL RATE AT EACH STAGE

80%
60%
40%
20%

PROSTATE
OVARY
PANCREAS
LUNG

STAGE I   STAGE II   STAGE III   STAGE IV

▼ **Some cancers can be too easy to find.** About 80 percent of prostate cancers are detected early. Yet most patients survive at least 5 years even if untreated. The problem: deciding whether medical intervention is necessary.

▼ **Other cancers are inherently elusive.** Pancreatic cancer, for one, betrays almost no symptoms, making diagnosis a matter of pure luck. Only 3 percent of cases are found in the first, most curable stage.

▼ **The money goes where the cancer is.** Some malignancies, notably lung cancer, are mostly detected only in late stages. As a result, that's where most research is directed. Shifting those priorities won't be easy.

lots of screening tests for lots of cancers. The promise of early detection is that it will be able to reveal a tumor before the tumor forms, that blood tests and next-generation imaging technologies will serve as surrogates for the human senses, just as Vesalius would have wanted. This new approach treats diagnosis as an algorithm, a sequence of calculations that can detect or predict cancer years before it betrays itself. It starts with a statistical screening that identifies the people, like Brenda Rosenthal, who have a greater risk of disease because of their genetics. Those people then periodically have a blood test that looks for specific proteins, or biomarkers, correlated to specific cancers (biomarkers can also be used to discriminate between dangerous and nonlethal cancers). Only with a positive blood test result does the algorithm shift to an imaging test, which is used to eliminate false positives and to isolate the location of a tumor in the body. The process is methodical, mathematical, and much more likely to find cancer than the current diagnostic procedures.

Statistics, though, beget statistics. For early detection of cancer to save lives, it will have to reliably identify those with a 90 percent chance of survival. The priorities of medical science should be not only to offer hope to those who know they have cancer but also to give faces and names and stories to the millions who are momentarily ignorant that they have it, too.

DON LISTWIN LEARNED about the survival curve for ovarian cancer after his mother, Grace, was diagnosed with the disease in 2000. Doctors had diagnosed her with a bladder infection—twice—and prescribed antibiotics. Not surprisingly, that treatment didn't work. By the time her doctor established that she had ovarian cancer, it was in stage IV and she was 12 months from her death.

Listwin, a onetime heir apparent to CEO John Chambers at Cisco Systems, says his impulse was to sue the doctor, the hospital, and anyone else who looked culpable. "I thought their incompetence had killed my mother," he says now. "But then I started staring at the survival rates, and I realized that if she had just been over here at [stage I or II], she'd be alive today." An electrical engineer by training, Listwin started to ask questions. Why does survival drop off so steeply? What happens in later-stage cancers that makes them so lethal? And most obviously, why can't we find the killer cancers early? "This looked like an emergent systems problem, a systems biology problem," he says, talking just like an engineer. "And it looked like an opportunity to engineer solutions."

Listwin, who says he was at Cisco during "the right 10 years," before the tech bubble burst, left the company in 2000 at age 41 with $100 million in the bank. Typically, people like Listwin—wealthy, philanthropic, and touched by cancer's ruthlessness—get on the cure bandwagon. They take the disease personally and try to defeat it, to destroy it. But after looking at the numbers, Listwin talked with Lee Hartwell, PhD, the 2001 Nobel laureate in medicine and president and director of the Fred Hutchinson Cancer Research Center in Seattle. Dr. Hartwell suggested that early detection was a largely untested strategy for reducing the number of cancer deaths, and Listwin was drawn to the opportunity. In 2004, with Dr. Hartwell on board as a science advisor, he created the Canary Foundation, a research group with the single goal of developing a battery of screening tests by 2015, starting with ovarian cancer and moving on to pancreatic, lung, and prostate cancers.

In fact, much of the meager improvement in cancer survival rates seen over the past 30 years can be attributed not to new chemotherapies or treatments but to early detection. Deaths from skin cancer, which is the most obvious neoplasia to diagnose and treat, have fallen by 10 percent. Since the Pap test became routine in the United States in the 1950s, cervical cancer deaths have fallen by 67 percent. There are tests for these diseases not because they are biologically different from other cancers, but because they occur in accessible parts of the body. It's neither difficult nor prohibitively expensive nor dangerous to swab a cervix. Other areas of the body, though—the ovaries, the pancreas—are less accessible and harder to monitor. Consequently, their malignancies, when they're finally found, are far more deadly.

Despite this proven advantage, early detection is an afterthought in cancer research. The pharmaceutical industry spends nearly $8 billion annually on cancer research, according to the International Union Against Cancer, most of it steered toward drug development and late-stage treatments. The major cancer foundations likewise spend lavishly on cure-based research. And the National Cancer Institute (NCI) spends just 8 percent of its budget on detection and diagnosis research, but nearly a quarter goes to treatment research.

Compared to these sums, Canary's $5 million annual budget scarcely registers. Yet Canary stands out in the cancer research community because its focus is on early detection rather than treatment. In effect, rather than getting snagged in the eddies of drug development and beneath the waterfalls of a cure paradigm, Canary headed upstream, away from the cancer cases that have faces on them and toward those that at least have a good shot at survival.

IN CASE THE ALLUSION ISN'T OBVIOUS, the Canary Foundation takes its name from the avian early detection system used by coal miners

Priorities in Cancer Research

In the $5 billion the National Cancer Institute spent in 2008, drug research was allotted nearly three times as much funding as early detection and diagnosis.

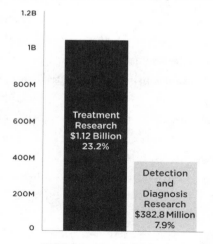

Treatment Research $1.12 Billion 23.2%

Detection and Diagnosis Research $382.8 Million 7.9%

SOURCE: National Cancer Institute; based on 2008 budget

to warn them of unsafe air. Listwin, whose year-round tan, golf-pro good looks, and cheerful swagger make him seem younger than his years, adopts the plumage of the namesake bird at every opportunity, wearing a canary yellow blazer to most foundation functions. Given his energetic manner, though, the yellow jacket brings to mind less a song-bird than a hornet, buzzing around and ever ready to engage.

Canary has recruited about 125 researchers who work at universi-ties and research institutes in the United States and Canada, all collabo-rating on creating a test in two parts—a blood test followed by an imaging test. This two-stage approach, Listwin hopes, will result in tests ready for clinical trial by 2015. Some researchers are engaged in pro-teomics—tracking down the proteins that could be used as markers for particular cancers. Others are developing imaging tools that can pin-point a tumor as small as 2 millimeters across (eschewing expensive technologies like CT scans, these new tools use cheaper technologies). Still others are designing the cost-benefit models that will help determine whether a test has commercial potential, given the available treatments. The Canary approach should sound familiar: It is in many ways a para-gon of smart screening, having one eye fixed on the bottom line and the other on the survival rate.

The 2015 milestone should raise some eyebrows. Such timetables, of course, are notoriously shaky—the NCI launched its war on cancer in 1971 with the objective of finding a cure within a decade, only to reset the goal in 1985 to cutting mortality in half by 2000, another missed target (the organization's current mission omits the word "cure" alto-gether). The Canary teams have been at their pursuit for 6 years rather than 40, but their goal is much more precise than something so grandi-ose as a cure. That makes their chances of success better, but it doesn't mean it's not still a numbers game.

II.

THOUGH I HAVEN'T USED THE TERM MUCH, this book has been filled with talk of biomarkers. Blood glucose is a biomarker for diabetes, cholesterol is a biomarker for heart disease, and genes and SNPs—single nucleotide polymorphisms—can be biomarkers for various diseases. Indeed, anything in the human body that can be measured and evaluated to indicate the presence for risk of a particular biological state counts as a biomarker.

Traditionally, biomarkers are used to either evaluate the state of the human body (are your liver enzymes within the normal range?) or to diagnosis a potential disease state (is your creatine kinase level high, indicating possible heart disease?). But a biomarker that is specific to a disease state—meaning that if it's there, you have the disease—is particularly valuable for early detection. These days, many diseases have been associated with potential biomarkers, from blood markers for stroke, to inflammation markers for gallstones or pancreatitis, to DNA markers for potential kidney disease. The hard part is turning a marker into a test.

The first significant biomarker to be associated with a specific kind of cancer came to light in 1965, with the discovery of carcinoembryonic antigen, or CEA. You probably read right over the word, but look at *carcinoembryonic* again and you'll see *carcino*, meaning "cancer," and *embryonic*, meaning "fetus." That odd combination is explained like this: CEA is a protein the body normally uses to build cells during fetal development. By the time we're born, we stop producing CEA. Except, it turns out, when we get certain kinds of cancer, mostly gastrointestinal cancers like those in the colon and stomach. As these cancers grow, CEA is thrown into the bloodstream, making its presence a useful (but far from foolproof) test for some kinds of cancer. A similar insight led to the discovery of PSA, the biomarker used to detect prostate cancer, in 1979. These discoveries were followed by more frustration than success in locating other cancer markers. But the past 10 years have seen a frenzy of ambitious research, with scientists embarking on dedicated hunts for the bloodborne trails of one disease or another.

In cancer, proteomics is among the most promising areas for biomarker research. If you thought the genome was complicated, consider the proteome, which encompasses all the proteins produced by a genome (and if there are 3 billion base pairs in our DNA, our proteome contains . . . well, nobody knows how many proteins). Proteins are the workhorses of our biology, the molecules that compose our muscles and nerves and connective tissues, the vessels that carry oxygen to our cells and carbon dioxide away from them, and the regulators that control how our organs function and how our bodies grow and repair.

It's in this last capacity that proteomics has potential as a tool for cancer detection. Since specific cells and organs rely on and produce specific proteins, the hunch is that cancer cells will release particular proteins that will turn up in the body only when a cancer emerges.

BACK WHEN CANARY first came together in 2004, proteomics was already on the map as a powerful tool for early detection. All the Canary teams needed to do, it seemed, was pump biomarkers through the testing process, identify the handful that link to early stage cancers, corroborate the results with a CT scan or MRI, and then roll out the early detection tests. "It looked like a pretty simple problem," says Patrick Brown, MD, PhD, a biochemist at Stanford and a member of Canary's ovarian cancer team.

Dr. Brown is one of those scientists of voracious appetites, whose curricula vitae can be parsed to tell any number of stories. Trained as a pediatrician, he's also a geneticist, and he pioneered the development of DNA microarrays. In his office, peeking out from under piles of books and papers, you'll find boxes of Lego Mindstorms kits, relics of an idea he had for building a robot probe. A deeply skeptical scientist, Dr. Brown functions at Canary as something like a bug tester, probing for logical flaws, false assumptions, and overly wishful thinking. Yet even he, early on, thought the science was all there for the taking. "Get a molecule, make a test, and you're done. It was just a matter of going out and finding them."

Dr. Brown doesn't think that anymore. "It's gone from something that seems really simple and really boring scientifically," he says, "to something that's not at all simple and, therefore, really compelling scientifically." The complications that have turned up in researching blood protein biomarkers, he says, are riddles that must be solved before the way forward becomes clear. And two riddles stand out.

The first goes something like this: In the past decade, proteomics has been great at discoveries—those eureka moments when proteins are identified and strongly associated with cancers. The field has identified thousands of proteins in cancerous human tissue, and hundreds of research papers have claimed there are strong correlations between particular new markers and certain types of cancer. But there's been a dearth of validation—the more laborious process of confirming the results and establishing that a protein appears consistently enough to use it as a biomarker for a particular cancer and that it isn't the result of some other condition like inflammation or anxiety.

The problem starts with the very structure of proteomic investigation. Most of these are case-control studies, in which proteins extracted from known cancer patients (the cases) are compared with proteins extracted from healthy volunteers (the controls). In a perfect study, the cases and the controls are matched up in every way—age, sex, diet, hometown—except for the fact that half of the sample has cancer. That way, any differences that turn up are statistically likely to be due to the cancer. But in reality, good samples of cancer tissue are in short supply, so most research is done in a take-what-you-can-get mode. The controls are assembled afterward, matching them to the cases as closely as possible. The result is that the cases and controls often have little in common—they can be of different ages or come from different towns or differ from each other in countless other variables. "So it's not surprising that you find all sorts of differences between the cases and controls," says Dr. Hartwell. "But those differences could have nothing whatsoever to do with the fact that they have cancer."

Take the case of prolactin. In 2008, a research group at Yale announced that it had identified several biomarkers that together could work as a test for ovarian cancer. (More markers mean better odds of a true positive, since different people have different proteins in their blood at different times.) The Yale markers included CA-125; osteopontin, a protein believed to be overexpressed in several cancers; and prolactin, a pituitary hormone found in the breasts, ovaries, and other organs. A test for early detection of ovarian cancer that was based on these biomarkers was released commercially by LabCorp in June 2008 under the name OvaSure.

The test troubled the Canary ovarian team, which had already taken stock of a few of these and other markers and ruled them insufficient for a valid test. The inclusion of prolactin, in particular, stood out. "It looked wrong to me," says Nicole Urban, ScD, cohead of women's cancer research at the Fred Hutchinson cancer center. "It seemed highly unlikely that it was related to the cancer."

So Dr. Urban ran her own study, comparing prolactin levels in women with ovarian cancer to those who were cancer free. She also made sure to track other variables: when and under what circumstances the blood was drawn. It turned out that when blood was drawn for a routine blood test, prolactin was present in normal levels in cases and controls alike. But the level spiked dramatically when blood was drawn right before a patient went into surgery—whether it was surgery for ovarian cancer or another procedure. In other words, Dr. Urban concluded, prolactin isn't a biomarker for cancer, it's a biomarker for a stressed-out patient about to go under the knife. (In October 2008, after the Food and Drug Administration warned that there were "serious regulatory problems" with the OvaSure test, LabCorp withdrew it from the market. The conflict did not involve the test's effectiveness.)

The ambiguity about prolactin's status as a biomarker exemplifies the leap required to get from an apparent signal to a true signal. "A good biomarker will tell us something we don't know," says Martin McIntosh, PhD, of the Fred Hutchinson cancer center, who crunched the prolactin numbers with Dr. Urban. "But even worse is when you think you have a good biomarker, and it's telling us something we don't actually want to know." And that's the first riddle of biomarkers.

But assume that science eventually makes that leap and a list of biomarkers with proven links to specific cancers is in hand. The next step is to find these markers in the blood. This is the second riddle: It's one thing to find a biomarker in the research lab, using tissue known to be cancerous. But putting a test into clinical practice means you have to find the marker when it's floating around in the body, diluted in human blood. Doing that accurately and consistently is a far more daunting proposition.

Dr. Brown first noted this problem in a presentation at Canary's 2007 Early Detection Symposium. He started by laying out the yardsticks. The basic premise of early detection is that there's a window of opportunity when a would-be lethal cancer is germinating but potentially curable. For ovarian cancer, Dr. Brown put this window at about 4 years from the cancer's first stirrings. Assuming annual or biannual screening, an effective test, then, must be able to detect a cancer when it's too small to be lethal but large enough for a significant number of proteins to spill into the bloodstream. This boils down to a question of signal versus noise: Are the current testing technologies, known as assays, sensitive enough to catch those few extra molecules, or will they be lost amid the torrent of proteins?

Dr. Brown offered some preliminary calculations. He started by estimating the size of a pre-advanced-stage ovarian tumor during this window of opportunity. On average, these tumors are just 2 millimeters in diameter and 4 milligrams in mass. "That's less than 1/10,000,000 of the mass of the average adult!" Dr. Brown noted. But with current assay technology, a tumor would have to be closer to 30 millimeters in diameter, he figured, to throw off enough biomarker molecules to exceed the levels in normal women and be reliably identifiable in the blood. And at that size, he acknowledged, most ovarian cancers have already metastasized, so detection at this point wouldn't be likely to save a life. According to these calculations, the prospects for blood-based early detection looked bleak.

For more than a year, Dr. Brown's presentation hung over the project. It seemed to expose a paradox at the very core of early detection: What use is a biomarker if it doesn't show up on a test until it's too late?

The Canary approach may be collaborative, but it's also competitive. Sanjiv Sam Gambhir, MD, PhD, the head of Stanford's molecular imaging program and a Canary leader, had been working on a mathematical model to address the problem. Though Dr. Gambhir's specialty is radiology and imaging, his PhD is in mathematics, and he thought some additional number crunching might point the way. His model re-created the human bloodstream and sent some CA-125, the known marker for ovarian cancer, into the mix. Soon enough, Dr. Gambhir had his answer: According to his calculations, a blood test for a biomarker like CA-125 can reveal a growth as small as 0.5 millimeter, "maybe even $\frac{1}{10}$ of 1 millimeter," says Dr. Gambhir, who published his calculations in *PLoS Medicine*. "So it's not out of the question to have a blood test that can detect a tumor that's very small, small enough to work for early detection."

In other words: The riddle could be solved. A biomarker test is possible. Cancer can be detected.

THE USUAL WAY TO USE BIOMARKERS is to extract them from the body, typically by drawing a blood sample. But what if we took the opposite approach, leaving the biomarker inside the body and sending something inside to find it? "What we want are spies," says Dr. Gambhir. "We want molecular spies within the body."

Dr. Gambhir's spies go hand in hand with a new technology he's been developing at Stanford, an approach to imaging that counters many of the problems with CT scans discussed in the last chapter. Dr. Gambhir's specialty is molecular imaging, which involves going beyond the beautiful images of our insides—the results of anatomical imaging methods like CT scans and MRIs—and looking even deeper, to the molecular level. The idea behind molecular imaging is to inject just such spies into patients in the forms of chemicals primed to interact with specific tumors. On a scan, these chemicals will show up like lighthouses in a fog, pinpointing a specific tumor down to the millimeter.

Dr. Gambhir developed his spy strategy using positron-emission tomography (PET) scans, a form of radiation akin to an x-ray. With an injection of glucose—yes, sugar—a PET scan can reveal specific tumors and their locations. But a PET scan, which typically is done in combination with a CT scan, is terrifically expensive. So Dr. Gambhir has developed another approach that uses an imaging technology that's already cheap, ubiquitous, and easy to use: ultrasound. Many doctors' offices have a machine; you can even buy one for home use for a few thousand dollars (something most radiologists would caution against).

Ultrasound, of course, has been around for decades, and we're all familiar with the blurry images of what we're told is a baby inside a mother's womb. But Dr. Gambhir's lab has crafted a way to transform ultrasound from a relatively imprecise tool that displays general anatomical information into a precise one that can discern details on the molecular level. First, the patient is injected with a chemical agent designed to seek out and attach to specific proteins on the surface of a tumor. Each of the molecules in this chemical agent is, in turn, attached to a microscopic bubble—a microbubble. When an ultrasound wand is swept over the body, the microbubbles vibrate, showing up on the ultrasound monitor as a sharp image. In animal studies, the technique can pinpoint a tumor as small as 2 millimeters. "It converts an anatomical tool into a molecular tool," Dr. Gambhir explained to me. What's more, it's cheap, because it piggybacks on an already common and inexpensive imaging technology. Dr. Gambhir and his colleagues at Stanford are now testing the technique on humans.

Dr. Gambhir presented his microbubble technique to his Canary colleagues at an ovarian cancer team retreat in Montana, at the vacation home of Don Valentine, a legendary venture capitalist who also happens to be Listwin's father-in-law. Standing beneath a massive buffalo head mounted over the fireplace in the log house's living room, Dr. Gambhir explained how the microbubble technique is significantly more promising than CT scans because the microbubbles can be primed to fix on only the tumors deemed to be most dangerous, rather than revealing just any unusual growth. "It shows us what we want," Dr. Gambhir said, speaking in the dry monotone of a scientist. "It's tumor-specific information at the molecular level."

Listwin was ecstatic. "This is a big deal," he said eagerly, his excitement contrasting with Dr. Gambhir's more clinical tone. "This is the beauty of a two-stage test. You don't go from screening to scalpel. You've got to have stage two. And that's what Sam has here."

III.

IF YOU DIED 50 YEARS AGO, your body stood a pretty good chance of serving science. In the 1940s, autopsy rates at US hospitals exceeded 50 percent. Pathologists weren't necessarily looking for what killed people, they were taking advantage of the fact that a body was available and ready for inspection. Like Vesalius, they were eager to learn about the human condition. There was still much to learn about how our bodies work, the thinking went, so every corpse was an educational opportunity.

These days, autopsy rates have fallen to below 10 percent, and that decline is symptomatic of a larger, unfortunate trend. Medicine has become all about finding a problem—a tumor, a heart attack, a failing kidney—and attacking it. It's all about the cure. Along the way, it has given up on measuring and tracking the basics. It has forgotten about normal. And not knowing normal may be the most important problem of all.

Knowing normal means knowing the basic state of the human body, so that we can understand whether something that looks wrong really *is* wrong. In science, they call this the baseline, a neutral state that serves as a basis for comparing whether later changes are significant divergences or simply normal variations. The Human Genome Project is an example of seeking to know normal, an effort to create a "reference genome" that can be compared with future variations. And on a personal level, learning our genetic makeups by using one of the personal-genomics services discussed in Chapter 3 would be a way of assessing our own baseline states.

What's normal does turn up here and there: A lab report, for example, will list a stream of normal ranges for this or that blood test. But considering that comparison to the baseline is a well-known principle, normal is given surprisingly short shrift these days, even though scientists are often confronted by their lack of baseline knowledge. Indeed, it's surprising how many areas of medical research lack a basic understanding of what's normal.

Take the role of fat in the human body. Until just a few years ago, fat, or adipose tissue, as it's technically called, was understood simply as a passive repository of extra calories in the body. But now it seems that the accumulation of fat also causes hormonal changes that affect the immune system. Fat can act almost like an organ, having significant influence on metabolism. But just how it works isn't well understood. Similarly, the immune system itself is a poorly understood and under-studied factor in our health, playing a black-box sort of role in inflam-matory conditions like Crohn's disease. For that matter, scant little is known about how cancer actually progresses in the human body; the "natural history of disease," as it's referred to, is a largely unresearched phenomenon. And then there are questions that you'd think medicine would have answered long ago, such as how many cells there are in a human body (estimates range from 1 trillion to several trillion), to the number of proteins in our blood (answers vary from 50,000 to millions), to the basic question of how many people in the world die from what causes (remarkably, not even the World Health Organization has a sound grasp of these numbers, and the Bill and Melinda Gates Foundation, among others, is trying to collect better data).

Part of this aversion to studying what's normal relates to the CT scan and other imaging tools discussed in Chapter 6. The scans are great at finding things, but what things? Many are what doctors call "inciden-talomas," smudges that look like cancer but are discovered, often after surgery, to be benign. And then there's the question of just what sorts of tumors need treatment in the first place, a nagging problem with pros-tate and other slow-growing cancers. The truth is, our bodies are devel-oping cancer cells all the time, and nearly all the time, our immune systems successfully fight them off.

It seems like it should be easy just to step back and survey the broad picture. But research costs money, and studying what's normal is gener-ally considered trivial, dismissed as "butterfly collecting," a diverting but inconsequential waste of time. At the National Institutes of Health (NIH), for instance, all grants are given "priority scores," indications of the projects' novelty, originality, and "scientific merit." Normal need not apply. Even the structure of the NIH dissuades studying normal; even though the *H* stands for "Health," most of its 27 separate institutes are organized around diseases, from the National Institute of Allergy and Infectious Diseases to the National Institute of Arthritis and Musculo-skeletal and Skin Diseases to the National Institute on Drug Abuse. Only the lowly National Institute of General Medical Sciences is tasked with "basic biomedical research that is not targeted to specific diseases." With a budget of $1.9 billion, it gets roughly one-third the funding that the NCI does, and just 6 percent of the overall NIH budget.

But in these data-rich days, studying what's normal could be a project of startling originality and merit. With petabytes of storage and ample processing power at hand, there's an opportunity to create a sort of Normal Human Project—a macro understanding of human biology on a micro scale. Or, as Dr. Brown describes it, a "comprehensive, quantitative molecular and cellular characterization of the normal human."

But even if it's not a popular concept at the NIH, normal is gaining ground among technology folks. At Microsoft, Jim Karkanias, senior director of applied research and technology, has been working on a software system called Amalga Life Sciences, a data-crunching tool that Karkanias calls a "database of experience." Conceivably, he says, there should be no limit on the amount of data that we pull from ordinary life, and no limit to the insights it might offer in return. "If you collect all the pieces of data on a human being, you can start to create what this normal baseline might be," he says. "This lets me collect as much data as I possibly can and then see what I can make of it. We call it the reference architecture for humans." Among the first customers for Amalga, not surprisingly, is Dr. Lee Hartwell's Fred Hutchinson Cancer Research Center.

Studying normal requires a rare combination of humility and audacity. First, scientists must acknowledge how much they don't know, and then they have to go off and create staggeringly complex computer systems to try to find the answers. But it's better than the alternative of assuming that, this time, we've got it all figured out. Time and again, when medicine presumes to have all the answers, the human body has shown itself to be a little more complicated than our neat and tidy explanations would have it be.

THE CANARY FOUNDATION HAS MADE "normal" a central part of its mission. In 2007, the team started the Baseline Program, an effort to quantify some basic metrics of human biology. Led by Dr. Brown and Dr. McIntosh, the Baseline Program group is focused on knowing normal in two areas: the normal range of gene expression in the healthy human body and the normal range and variation of proteins in the blood.

Gene expression is the process by which the information contained in our DNA kicks off a product, typically a protein. It's the dog responding to the command of its genetic master. The form of that expression depends on the need at hand; though our DNA remains the same throughout our bodies, it is expressed for different purposes at different places in our bodies. Using tissues taken from several locations in the body, Dr. Brown is attempting to map exactly what tissues express what genes. By identifying the normal range of expression in these tissues, Dr. Brown hopes to assemble a baseline that can be compared against any unusual gene expression signals in the body.

The protein effort involves cataloging the thousands of proteins that are present in healthy blood in a database that can be matched against a sample from someone with cancer in the hope of identifying unique and cancer-specific markers. The effort is paying off; Dr. McIntosh recently concluded that proteins vary widely from human to human but remain fairly consistent in any one person. That insight makes the case for having a proteomic profile done when we're young, so in later years it can be used as a baseline to pick up any new, worrisome signals that may come from a cancer.

Dr. McIntosh offers an analogy. "In World War II, the British army decided to put more armor plating on its airplanes. But they couldn't put it everywhere, because it would make the planes too heavy to fly; they only wanted to put the armor where it was needed. So the mechanics went out to the airfield and looked at where the bullet holes were in the planes." At this point the statistician pauses and smiles. "But then the statisticians came in," he continues. "'No,' they said. 'These are the planes that made it back. Don't put the armor where the bullet holes are. Put it where they aren't.'"

The analogy is this: It could be that cancers that are found early have a 90 percent survival rate not just because they're caught early but also because they're easier to catch. The most lethal cancers, on the other hand, are the ones that are especially hard to spot. We don't need biomarkers or imaging tests that reveal the cancers that are survivable. We need tests for the ones that are really going to kill us.

WHEN PRESIDENT BARACK OBAMA CALLED FOR "a cure for cancer in our time" in his February 2009 address to the US Congress, he strode distressingly close to repeating the sort of thinking that had failed once before. After all, the war on cancer circa 1971 saw cancer as a single disease—one hulking enemy that could be bombed into submission with chemotherapy. That war has failed because cancer isn't one disease, but rather many diseases, with many strains and forms. It's what's called heterogeneity. Heterogeneity is a factor not just with cancer but also with many other diseases that we now battle, from stroke to heart disease. But cancer may be the most diverse disease. Some cancer researchers put the total number of cancers at 200; others say it's thousands. Matched by $10 billion in new funding for the NIH for short-term stimulus purposes, Obama's call for curing a singular cancer may just have been a slip in syntax, a turning to the strongest sort of language to make his point. But his appeal for a "cure" indicates how resistant conventional wisdom is to the complicated reality of a condition that defies our best efforts to take it on.

The fact that cancer isn't one disease but many demonstrates both the challenge and the opportunity of the Canary approach. By starting at the opposite end of the disease chain from conventional research, the

Canary team is directing its intellectual and financial resources toward understanding the disease—its variations, progression, molecular characteristics—rather than focusing on the blunt instruments of chemotherapy and radiation. It's a route holding no small number of frustrations and dead ends. And it is by no means a route that promises, in the end, to actually succeed. But the approach has promise because it reflects the best practices of science. It approaches cancer as a biological system of great complexity, one that may be unique to every individual facing the disease. And rather than becoming beholden to any one biomarker, test, or treatment, the Canary philosophy is really about the platform, a flexible strategy that can scale across diseases. Change the disease, change the inputs, and the strategy is still sound: Match the right biomarkers to the right diseases. Create a two-stage test. And intervene early.

The challenges that linger in developing methods for the early detection of cancer reflect a larger disconnect between how we want medicine to work and how it actually does work. When we go to the doctor, we expect a definitive diagnosis—a true verdict of what's wrong. After getting that, we then expect a clear prognosis—an expert prediction of what's going to happen. And ultimately, we want our cure, our surefire route to return us to health.

But the thing is, no matter how brilliant your physician may be, these things always boil down to guesses—informed by lab tests and experience, perhaps, but still guesses. We want medicine to be deterministic, to follow clear laws and mechanisms. But in reality, it's almost always probabilistic, more calculation than divination. There is no certainty in medicine. Early detection, which is steeped in probability predictions and statistics, just makes these calculations more transparent than we're used to. Short of running a complete molecular breakdown of the human body (which remains impossible), early detection will always be a numbers game.

For a disease like cancer that is so often seen as a death sentence, early detection promises a trade-off. At first, it makes things more complicated. It introduces more doubt and complexity into an already complicated equation. But in return, early detection promises that this doubt can be quantified, that these new variables can be broken down into metrics, analyzed, and factored into our health decisions. Early detection proposes that the result of this calculation—complicated and ambiguous as it is—will yield better results for individuals and their families. In exchange for a modicum of doubt, it offers the maximum opportunity for hope.

PART III

Care and Treatment

A Little Drug Problem

Why Most Drugs Don't Work, and Why Finding Ones That Do Is So Hard

I.

IN 1961, A YOUNG SCIENTIST at the Naval Medical Research Institute in Bethesda, Maryland, stared at a glass jar and began to wonder. Inside the jar was a living rabbit thyroid gland; a few days earlier he had injected the gland with some cancer cells. As expected, a few tumors appeared on the gland. But looking inside the jar again, the 27-year-old scientist, whose name was Judah Folkman, MD, noticed that the tumors weren't growing. They stayed small, about the size of a pencil tip. And he couldn't imagine why.

It took about 10 years, but Dr. Folkman would eventually have his answer: The gland may have been alive, but without the rest of the rabbit attached, there was no blood supply to the thyroid. And without blood, the cancer couldn't grow. It was a startling insight, one that ran contrary to the conventional wisdom about how a tumor progresses. "Most research is failure," Dr. Folkman recalled later. "You go years and years and years, and then every once in a while there is a tremendous finding, and you realize for the first time in your life that you know something that hour or that day that nobody else in history has ever known, and you can understand something about how nature works."

Dr. Folkman's epiphany became known as angiogenesis, the theory that a tumor needs blood to grow. And it offered the corollary theory of anti-angiogenesis: the idea that if a tumor could be cut off from its blood supply, then it couldn't survive. Dr. Folkman first published the idea in a 1971 paper, but for years, few people in the world of cancer research actually took his theory seriously. It just seemed . . . wrong. "Tumor growth cannot be dependent upon blood vessel growth any more than infection is dependent upon pus," reviewers at the National Cancer Institute said in turning down Dr. Folkman's first grant application. That perception began to change in the 1980s, after researchers in his lab isolated one substance that indeed seemed to lure blood capillaries toward a new tumor. And in 1994, another researcher in Dr. Folkman's lab identified a substance that did the opposite: It seemed to inhibit blood vessels from growing. Dr. Folkman and his team called this substance angiostatin and started experiments in mice.

The results exceeded all expectations: Not only did the angiostatin cause tumors to stop growing, but when it was combined with a similar molecule called endostatin, the tumors would actually shrink and ultimately disappear altogether. Encouraged, Dr. Folkman licensed his research to EntreMed, a small biotech firm in Maryland. And in November 1997, Dr. Folkman's team published the results of its animal research in the science journal *Nature*. As word began to spread, Dr. Folkman's insight of nearly 40 years before seemed poised to finally bear fruit, and angiostatin and endostatin quickly became the most promising cancer drugs in the pharmaceutical pipeline. "We believe that [EntreMed] may have found the Achilles' heel of cancer," one financial analyst told potential investors in February 1998, urging them to buy the company's stock, and fast.

A few weeks later, *New York Times* reporter Gina Kolata was at a dinner party, where she had a conversation with James Watson, PhD, the Nobel laureate and codiscoverer of the DNA double helix. As any good reporter might, Kolata asked Dr. Watson if there was anything he was excited about. Judah Folkman's work, Watson said, describing it in glowing terms.

Six weeks later, on May 3, the front page of the *New York Times* featured a "Special Report" with the headline "Hope in the Lab." The story began: "Within a year, if all goes well, the first cancer patient will be injected with two new drugs that can eradicate any type of cancer, with no obvious side effects and no drug resistance—in mice." Angiostatin and endostatin, the story said, could "make tumors disappear and not return." For added oomph, Kolata quoted what Dr. Watson had told her at the dinner party: "'Judah is going to cure cancer in two years.'"

WHEN WE GET SICK, drugs are often the first things we think of: What can I take to get better? In this regard, drugs are more than mere molecules. Yes, we want the chemistry to work; we need these substances to accomplish the immediate task of salving pain or healing wounds. But drugs come preloaded with hopes and expectations. Every dose— whether it comes by pill or injection—packs the promise of a different prognosis, a new path. Drugs hint at a different life story.

In the past 50 years, modern pharmacology has created dozens of treatments that improve and save lives. Cardiovascular drugs like beta-blockers have drastically reduced deaths from heart attacks and heart disease. For every million people who take a statin drug for high cholesterol, there are 50,000 fewer angioplasties, surgeries, heart attacks, strokes, and cardiovascular deaths, studies have shown. And in the past 15 years, drugs have transformed AIDS from a death sentence into a

Hit and Miss Drugs

The truth is no drug works for everybody—and some don't even work for most.

Therapeutic Area	Efficacy Rate
Alzheimer's	30%
Asthma	60%
Diabetes	57%
Incontinence	40%
Migraine (acute)	52%
Rheumatoid arthritis	50%

SOURCE: *Physician's Desk Reference*

managed disease. These are just some of the triumphs of pharmacology, and each case is a bona fide miracle, a life transformed.

But not every drug can deliver a fairy-tale ending. Many of the stories we expect from drugs are partly fictions, hiding in a gauze of ambiguous results, placebo effects, and messy side effects. Though it's widely known that the pharmaceutical industry tests hundreds of substances to get the handful that work, most people assume that those that *are* approved by the Food and Drug Administration (FDA) are actually effective. But the numbers say otherwise.

Even the best drugs have imperfect chances of working for any one person. Asthma drugs work in about 60 percent of patients. Migraine drugs are effective in only about half of cases. Drugs for Alzheimer's disease work in about 30 percent of patients. And those are exceptional results compared to cancer drugs, which at best work about 25 percent of the time. What's more, these statistics are drawn from clinical trials— closely monitored research environments where all variables are controlled and patients are strictly monitored for compliance. In the real world, people are less dutiful, conditions are more chaotic, and drugs can be even more of a shot in the dark.

Consider, for instance, treatments for depression. Worldwide, antidepressant sales amount to more than $20 billion a year, making them among the most prescribed drugs in the world. But finding the right drug for the right patient is notoriously difficult and typically involves a long slog of trial and error. A few years ago, the National Institute of Mental Health (NIMH) launched a study known as the Sequenced Treatment Alternatives to Relieve Depression (STAR*D) study to examine exactly how patients experience antidepressants. As in real life, STAR*D treatments depended upon trial and error: Volunteers with clinical depression would take one drug after another, hoping to end up with one that helped.

Patients began STAR*D in level 1, where they were given citalopram, a widely prescribed antidepressant sold under the brand name Celexa. If after 12 to 14 weeks the patients didn't report significant improvement, they went to level 2, where they tried a different drug or therapy. And so on, through levels 3 and 4, until something worked.

So how did the drugs do in this real-world scenario? At the end of level 1, only one-third of patients reported that the first drug had alleviated their symptoms to the point of remission. Another 10 to 15 percent reported having some smaller effect, and 9 percent dropped out due to side effects. After 12 more weeks in level 2, a total of 50 percent of patients reported that their symptoms had been relieved; after all four levels, that total had climbed to about 70 percent. The NIMH called these results "particularly good," and indeed they fall within the range of what psychiatrists generally expect for antidepressants.

But step outside the industry, and the findings lead to quite another conclusion. In plain language, STAR*D found that if you're depressed, you could spend 3 months on a potent psychotropic drug and have only a 33 percent chance of getting relief. After almost 6 months on drugs, your chances of total relief could be bumped up to about fifty-fifty—a coin flip—and you risked side effects like sexual dysfunction, insomnia, and weight gain. The result is a $20 billion market for products that take 6 months to work half the time (and don't forget that antidepressants have a notoriously high placebo-effect rate of up to 50 percent, meaning that as many as half of the patients in a study who receive a sugar pill report that their depression gets better). That may be good odds for the industry, but it seems a poor bet for a patient.

The inconsistent effectiveness of today's drugs most likely goes back to the idea of heterogeneity of disease mentioned in Chapter 7. Just because we have a common name for a condition doesn't mean that there's only one thing going on within the body. What's collectively referred to as heart disease may in reality be tens or hundreds or some unknown multitude of actual root causes. What we call cancer has been more accurately carved up into many hundreds of types and subtypes— fast- and slow-growing carcinomas, early and late-stage lymphomas, hard- and soft-tissue sarcomas, and on and on. And at least these categories are based on actual biology. Psychiatric disorders are almost entirely opaque, with potentially hundreds or thousands of conditions being lumped into one bucket.

As far as science goes, heterogeneity is a good thing. It's something we want to understand with the hope that, eventually, those distinctions

A Decision Tree for Depression

In 2001, the National Institute of Mental Health began the landmark STAR*D study, which aimed to test antidepressants in a real-world scenario of trial and error through four levels of different drugs, a process that could take a year to complete. Seventy percent of those who went through all four levels reported success—but by that point, more than 40 percent of all participants had dropped out.

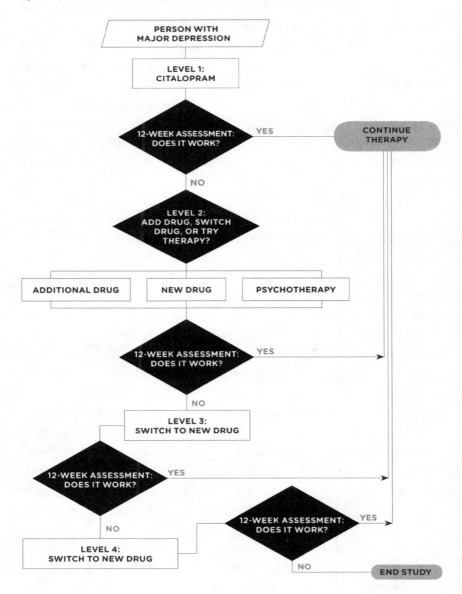

will allow for more precise treatments. But in the meantime, the profusion of disease types and causes means that drugs will remain imperfect instruments. They will work sometimes, for some people. The more conscious we are of this fact, the better prepared we will be for weathering what works and the inevitable disappointments along the way.

II.

THIS SHOULD BE A GOLDEN AGE for the drug business. Medical research has accomplished terrific things in the past 2 decades. The human genome has been decoded, opening the door to greater understanding of how drugs do their work. Bioinformatics—the combining of biological data with computing power—makes it possible to learn how diseases work in the body and find new drug targets. Computers are now able to create virtual models of how various molecules work inside the body, potentially shortening the actual time that will be needed to sort through molecules in a lab. And the new science of systems biology can offer us a comprehensive understanding of the complexity that goes on inside us, flushing out possible toxic reactions and side effects far earlier than before.

But despite these advances, the day-to-day reality has been a disappointment, full of false starts and dead ends. High throughput screening, in which hundreds of thousands of compounds are combined with a protein to look for a spark that might signal a promising treatment, has turned up lots of noise but scarce signals. Meanwhile, the pipeline of new drugs has slowed to a crawl, as one promising candidate after another has petered out in the last phases of development. "The low-hanging fruit has been picked," says Derek Lowe, PhD, a drug discovery chemist and industry pundit.

Some experts consider this not a science problem so much as a business problem. William Haseltine, PhD, a former researcher at Harvard Medical School and the founder of Human Genome Sciences and eight other biotechnology companies, casts a cold eye on the blockbuster model itself. "The need for a blockbuster is ineluctable," he says, noting that fewer than 1 in 100 new ideas reaches clinical trials and fewer than 10 percent of these are approved for sale. "What science can deliver is pretty clear. Usually you can predict the consequences of a trial, you can see what the pathway of a drug is going to be. These days, they're working very narrow pathways, and you can do a reasonably rapid test on a small number of people and get something through the FDA.

"The problem is," he continues, "that these companies' structures won't allow these smaller drugs to reach the market. These are usually $50 [million] to $100 million markets, and that's not big enough. So they'll alter the process to try to create a bigger drug, and that becomes a recipe for failure. If you insist that a drug reaches $1 billion or more in sales, very few drugs will do that. And if you try to make it do that, the drug will probably fail."

Dr. Haseltine does have a solution for this bipolar disorder within the pharmaceutical industry. He suggests that drug companies separate their research arms from their marketing arms. Let the scientists pursue the science, and let the marketers sell the results. He draws an analogy with the way the computer industry runs along two channels: The technology for faster processors or smarter touchscreens gets created by small companies, who then sell it to the large brands, who figure out how to package it and exploit the results.

Truth be told, though, he doesn't actually expect the drug companies to do this. "They're unwilling to make the major changes in the research and development," he says of big drug companies like Pfizer and GlaxoSmithKline. "They're locked into this huge marketing-driven infrastructure already." Rather, he says, the opportunity is for new companies to create a different model of drug development altogether. Dr. Haseltine imagines that smaller groups—often spun out of university labs—will each work on their own drugs, outsourcing the chemical discovery, the screening, and the trials. These could be aggregated into 20 or 30 or 40 smaller teams and managed by larger drug discovery companies. The best candidates, including those drugs with merely $50 million markets, would then be sold off to drug marketing companies.

From the industry's point of view, part of the riddle here is that drug development is a race against the clock. A US patent lasts for 20 years, and since the United States is usually the biggest market for any drug, a pharma company needs to file for a patent as soon as a promising molecule is isolated and ready for trials. At that point, the clock starts ticking away, even though there are years of trials ahead. In general, this system has worked for both the drug industry and the greater good. Patents strike a fair balance between, on the one hand, the inducements of profit—encouraging companies to put millions of dollars into research in exchange for a temporary monopoly on their discoveries—and the needs of society, which benefits once a patent expires and a drug becomes free for others to manufacture and improve upon.

That's the bright side of how intellectual property is protected in the drug business. But there's a dark side, found in the 99 out of 100 ideas that are left on the lab bench. Many of those molecules and therapies may well be unworthy of the drug company's time. But that's not to say they're not worth *somebody's* time. Dr. Haseltine is right when he decries the idea that because a drug doesn't represent a $1 billion market, it's not worth pursuing. All those discoveries being thrown in some drawer somewhere—becoming what I call dark data—is a travesty, a true case of science squandered. Not only are the dead ends of one company potentially instructive to another in the sense that they might prevent others from traveling down those same dead ends, but there might in fact be a financial model that makes a sub-billion-dollar market work. This is the shame of dark data, that one company's failures are treated as corporate secrets worthy of the same protections as its successes. That's all well and good for Nabisco or the software industry, but in the matter of drugs, where the bottom line is life and death, it's a travesty.

Dr. Haseltine believes this will soon change—not out of altruism, but because of economics. In the next decade, as big pharma companies run out of blockbuster drugs, they will discover that their old research has some value to others. "They'll start selling their old research portfolios: their hits, their leads, their phase I and phase II results," Dr. Haseltine predicts. And by doing so, they'll provide opportunities for others to make profits on lesser-selling drugs.

How a Drug Gets Approved

It typically takes a drug company 8 to 10 years and $1 billion to turn a promising chemical into an approved drug treatment. Here's how it happens.

Pre-clinical development

Thousands of molecules are identified and isolated in pharmaceutical industry labs, and the most promising drugs are tested in animals. Of these, only a fraction prove good enough to continue on to human testing.
1% chance of success

Phase I trials

Testing in humans begins, and promising drugs are tested for toxic side effects and targeting (which part of the body is affected). In most cases, effectiveness is not a goal of phase I trials.
20% chance of success

Phase II trials

In this stage, promising drugs are finally tested for efficacy in humans. Subjects are randomly assigned to a drug or a placebo, and the studies are double-blinded, meaning neither the subject nor the researchers know who is on the drug or the placebo. Dosages and response rates are monitored for signs of effectiveness.
30% chance of success

Phase III trials

In this most-expensive stage of testing, a drug is tested in several centers at once, again in randomized, double-blind trials.
60% chance of success

Submit to FDA for approval
75% chance of success

Approval

After an average of 10 months, the FDA will decide whether or not to approve the drug.

Source: Joe Northrup, "The Pharmaceutical Sector," in *The Business of Healthcare Innovation*, ed. Lawton Robert Burns.

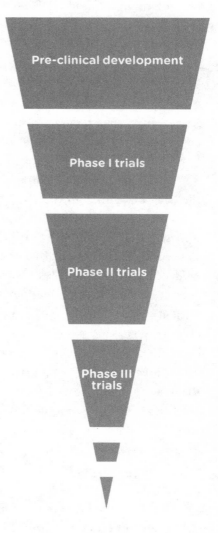

THE DRUG INDUSTRY'S HIGH FAILURE RATE also means that the few drugs that do get through the gauntlet of clinical trials and FDA approval become must-win propositions. With only a few years of patent protection left by that time, a company must pull out all the stops to sell the drug. This, once again, means marketing.

The drug industry excels at turning marketing dollars into prescriptions. The process starts with presentations and advertisements to doctors, who are pitched the promise that this new drug beats the old ones. Soon enough, prescriptions start to follow. This obscene marketing to physicians has been well covered elsewhere. Direct-to-consumer advertising is also driving demand for new treatments. But it's worth noting here that some marketing is designed to push out perfectly worthwhile older treatments (whose patent protection has often expired and can therefore be sold as cheap generics) in order to advance newer treatments (which *are* under patent protection, and therefore are more expensive).

But are the new drugs really better? The FDA doesn't require comparative clinical trials, only proof that the drug beats a placebo. So unless somebody were to compare drugs head to head, it's almost impossible to say. That was the premise behind the landmark ALLHAT study: Do side-by-side comparisons of various treatments for high blood pressure in order to see, once and for all, what the best treatment really is. When ALLHAT (short for Antihypertensive and Lipid-Lowering Treatment to Prevent Heart Attack Trial) began in 1994, the use of diuretics and beta-blockers was in decline, while three newer treatments—calcium channel blockers, angiotensin-converting enzyme inhibitors (known as ACE inhibitors), and alpha-adrenergic blockers—were on the rise. But since these newer drugs had only been compared to placebo when working their way to FDA approval, there was no way to know which treatment worked best.

The study, which recruited 42,000 individuals with elevated blood pressure, was one of the most ambitious ever carried out for the condition. The subjects were divided into four groups and given one of four treatments: a diuretic, an ACE inhibitor, a calcium channel blocker, or an alpha blocker. Within a few years, the alpha blocker arm of the trial was stopped: Patients were showing a 25 percent *increased* risk of heart disease. The other 30,000 patients continued their protocols for 5 years, and then the results were analyzed.

Published in 2002 and elaborated upon in 2006, the results were a disaster for the drug industry. Not only was the alpha blocker deemed too suspect to use, but the calcium antagonist and the ACE inhibitor both fell short of the cheap, common, and old-fashioned diuretic in lowering blood pressure and reducing the risk of heart disease. Patients on the newer, patented drugs had higher rates of stroke and heart failure.

The researchers could hardly contain their glee. "It's one thing to say we have new drugs and they're a little bit better, but I think this should really cause us to stop and think about defining what 'better' means in terms of real outcomes and not sales pitches," Robert Califf, MD, a cardiologist at Duke Medicine and a member of the ALLHAT Data and Safety Monitoring Board, said when the results became public. "The real news here is, who knows what other inexpensive generic drugs that are actually better are not being used because there's no one out there selling them to doctors?"

III.

THERE'S NO DOUBT THAT ASPIRIN is something of a magic bullet. Acetylsalicylic acid, as aspirin is technically known, works by blocking prostaglandins—powerful chemicals in the body that cause swelling and inflammation. Since prostaglandins also cause blood to clot, small doses of aspirin have been found to reduce the risk of stroke and heart attack (millions of people take them every day for this purpose). Aspirin has also been found to slow the progress of some forms of dementia, and it could reduce the risk of Alzheimer's disease. It even suppresses estrogen levels in women, reducing the risk of breast cancer.

It's been said, though, that had Bayer compounded the first stable form of aspirin yesterday, rather than 110 years ago, it would never get FDA approval. The problem is twofold: For one, aspirin doesn't really work like a magic "bullet" at all; it's more like a shotgun, having scattered effects on many different systems within the body. This is contrary to the current industry preference for drugs that work like bullets, hitting single, precise targets. And second, aspirin has long been known to come with side effects. It can cause serious gastric bleeding in some people, and it can cause Reye's syndrome, a potentially fatal neurological disease, in children. These side effects would be red flags to today's drug developers.

Tylenol, though, would have it even worse. Derived from coal tar, acetaminophen, the active chemical in Tylenol, was first introduced into medical practice in the 1880s. It was used sporadically until the 1950s, when Tylenol was introduced and marketed as being safer than aspirin because it was suitable for children and was easier on the stomach. The pitch worked, and Tylenol became the best-selling health product in the United States, with higher sales than Crest toothpaste. Today, acetaminophen is the most widely used pain reliever in the world.

But acetaminophen can be a profoundly dangerous drug. For some people, it is pure poison. Acetaminophen is the most common cause of liver failure in the United States, where about 50 percent of cases are attributed to acetaminophen toxicity, according to a 2005 study. This risk has been well known for more than a decade and has generally been associated with failing to follow the directions, taking too much acetaminophen, or combining the pain reliever with alcohol. In June 2009, an FDA advisory panel recommended that because of these dangers, drugs that combine acetaminophen and narcotics, such as Vicodin and Percocet, be removed from the market and that the maximum dose of acetaminophen be lowered.

But just a few weeks earlier, another, less celebrated red flag had been raised about the drug. In May 2009, researchers from the University of North Carolina in Chapel Hill and the Jackson Laboratory in Bar Harbor, Maine, suggested that in some people who suffered liver failure after taking the drug, the cause may be genetic, not the size of the dose.

The researchers found that in as many as one-third of healthy individuals, even a normal dose of acetaminophen dangerously raised blood levels of alanine transferase, a liver enzyme, suggesting damage to the liver. The researchers found that a single-letter (or SNP) variation on a gene known as *CD44* was significantly associated with liver injury. "The reality is that there is no safe drug," said Paul Watkins, a coauthor of the study. "Good drugs are bad for some people. Because different people respond differently to drugs, where you draw the line is not exactly black and white."

THE IDEA OF MATCHING DRUGS with our genes is known as pharmacogenomics. By isolating the relationship between particular drugs and particular genes, the theory goes, the right drug can be given to the right person at the right dose.

Pharmacogenomics has three main strategies. The first is to maximize efficacy by matching people up with the drug that works best for them. This is the rationale behind Gleevec (imatinib), a drug that treats a kind of leukemia known as chronic myelogenous leukemia, or CML. Gleevec is remarkably effective for CML, with 53 out of 54 patients in one study responding to the drug. Five-year survival rates for CML improved from about 30 percent before Gleevec to nearly 90 percent in patients who use it. The drug works so well because CML is a very specific disease caused by a single aberrant protein on a specific chromosome. Gleevec works by targeting that protein and nothing else.

The second strategy of pharmacogenomics is to minimize toxic effects by weeding out people who might have a specific vulnerability to a drug. The link between the *CD44* gene and acetaminophen is one example of this approach.

And the third approach is to use somebody's genetic makeup to fix a proper dose at the outset of treatment. The standout example here is warfarin, a drug used to prevent blood clots in people at risk for stroke. Too much warfarin can lead to excessive bleeding, while too little leaves a risk of clots and stroke—making it essential to find each patient's correct dose as quickly as possible. In early 2009, a team from Stanford University showed that variants of two genes could affect how the body processes warfarin. The team then created an algorithm that modified a patient's dose based on these variations. The algorithm homes in on the ideal dose, eliminating much of the usual trial and error.

Warfarin and Gleevec are the most prominent examples of pharmacogenomics success. But considering all the hype that pharmacogenomics has prompted over the past decade, they are rather lonely examples;

as of 2009, fewer than 20 drugs had been convincingly matched up with specific genetic variants, allowing physicians to modify treatments accordingly. For a research branch that's been hailed as the Rosetta stone of personalized medicine, this is thin pickings. Part of the reason for the slow pace is that the science, as so often happens, has proven more difficult than expected.

But there's also been a decided reticence on the part of the pharmaceutical industry to buy into pharmacogenomics. As Dr. Haseltine points out, the industry's blockbuster model likes big markets, not niches. The drug industry has gotten hooked on the big breakthroughs that pull in big markets that go on for years. Think Claritin for allergies, Prilosec for heartburn, Lipitor for high cholesterol—these drugs bring in billions of dollars annually for their manufacturers. Never mind the fact that something like Claritin barely works better than a placebo pill. The great appeal of these drugs is that they are used by a great number of people, including many who receive little or no benefit from them. The model here is similar to how people use ketchup—a whole lot more gets poured out of the bottle than necessary. This is the model that has propelled the industry to record profits over the past 2 decades, not going after a long tail of diseases and niche treatments.

So as we wait for pharmacogenomics to bear fruit, both economically and in terms of treatments, how do we make better decisions about which drugs we should take? How do we avoid the anguish of trial and error? Part of the answer lies in simply making it easier to understand what drugs are for and how they work. Better information, such as the Drug Facts box being considered by the FDA (see Chapter 1), would be a big help. These simple tools would help people understand what a drug is for, how effective it can be, and what the potential side effects are, because they'd be stated clearly and boldly. There are other decision aids on the Internet, tools that help patients match up their symptoms with a range of treatment options. At the moment, these mainly exist for conditions that demand elaborate drug management regimens, such as multiple sclerosis and diabetes. But the need for others is plain.

Perhaps the best model here is Adjuvant!, an online decision tool for physicians treating patients with cancer. *Adjuvant treatment* is the medical term for the therapies (typically chemotherapy with drugs or radiation therapy) used in cancer patients following surgery. The principle is that using a combination of treatments in a well-considered regimen will yield better results than surgery or chemotherapy alone. The trick, though, is knowing what that exact combination should be.

In the mid-1990s, Peter Ravdin, MD, PhD, an oncologist then at the University of Texas at San Antonio, realized that his hospital had assembled a wealth of information about how different drugs worked for different types of breast cancer, depending on a cancer's stage, the tumor's size, the patient's age, and so on. But because that information was locked up in a database, physicians had a difficult time connecting that data to their patients. Dr. Ravdin decided to create a computer program to do that, and he called it Adjuvant!

Adjuvant! is a fairly straightforward tool. A physician logs on and fills in a dozen fields using a patient's pathology report. The software crunches the numbers and delivers a printout of charts that lay out the risks and benefits of various therapies following surgery. It estimates the odds of death or relapse as well as the risks of possible side effects. The result connects the research with the patient, and this lets a doctor and the patient create a more informed treatment plan, as well as a more realistic prognosis.

Here's the catch: Adjuvant! is for physicians only. "The interpretation of some of the prognostic and staging information for any given person's case can be difficult even for an experienced professional," the Web site explains, adding that there is also a concern that "someone reviewing their prognosis alone . . . may find the information emotionally overwhelming." That warning aside, though, there's nothing stopping patients armed with their pathology reports from logging on and *saying* they're doctors.

Despite its physician-only approach, Adjuvant! is a model of Decision Tree thinking: It puts science within reach, it reorients it to personal circumstances, and it turns data into actionable information. For women with breast cancer, it's an awesome tool. But there are many other people who also need specific guidance on drugs. The real goal, then, would be for more innovators to take up Dr. Ravdin's lead and create other tools that people—not just physicians—could use to make smart choices about drugs.

The magic bullets allowed by pharmacogenomics will be wonderful, but there's a lot of science to do between here and there. In the meantime, there is a great deal that science already knows about how well we do on drugs and what drugs work for which people. Some of this information, of course, is kept locked up by the drug companies. But the opportunity remains there. Tailoring drugs to people doesn't always demand genetics; we can make the most of what we have even now.

The problem with magic bullets is that as often as they're miracles, they're illusions—or they're dangerous. As much as we may hope for miracle drugs, the reality is that they are few and far between.

IV.

THE FRONT-PAGE STORY in the *New York Times* about Judah Folkman's discoveries set off a firestorm. On the morning the story appeared, the stock price of EntreMed, which held the rights to angiostatin and endostatin, shot up fast. By the end of the day, shares were trading for $85 apiece, a sevenfold increase from the $12 per share they started the day at. Patients began clamoring for the drugs—they wanted them *now*. Some even traveled to EntreMed's Maryland headquarters to be first in line (they were politely turned away).

But the hype soon turned sour. Within days, James Watson, whose glowing quote about "curing cancer" probably did the most to hype EntreMed, wrote a letter to the *Times* claiming he had been misquoted. "The history of cancer research is littered with promised treatments that raised people's hopes," he wrote, "only for them to be dashed when the treatments were put to the test in humans." The National Cancer Institute backed away from the drugs, saying that it could not reproduce the results that Dr. Folkman's team had reported in *Nature* a few months before (they later did validate his research). And Dr. Folkman, who was reportedly deeply embarrassed by the *Times* story and the ensuing controversy, tried to get back to work in his lab. Meanwhile, as EntreMed's stock price returned to earth, the company began the years-long process of testing the drugs in phase I clinical trials.

For patients, though, the appeal of these drugs remained, and getting into an EntreMed trial became nothing short of winning a lottery: Thousands of patients asked to participate, although there were just 90 slots. Phase I trials began in early 1998. Patients received infusions of the drugs for 4 weeks, followed by several months of self-administered injections. After 2 years, the first phase of testing was complete. Endostatin and angiostatin suggested some promise. The drugs showed no toxicity (the main research interest in a phase I trial is safety), and some tumors seemed to stabilize or even shrink. But the effects were small, and far from what had been reported in mice. Phase II trials on the drugs began in 2002, but within a few months EntreMed decided the evidence was going the wrong way. That November, the company announced it would stop manufacturing the drug (it did agree to produce enough to complete the trials). In 2004 it transferred ownership of the drugs back to Dr. Folkman's hospital.

By this time, though, angiogenesis was no longer considered Dr. Folkman's folly. Several other labs had begun research into the theory, including Genentech, a biotechnology company in Silicon Valley. Genentech had been pursuing its own lead since 1989, when scientist Napoleone Ferrara, MD, isolated a substance in cow pituitary glands called vascular endothelial growth factor, or VEGF. The substance appeared to encourage blood vessels to grow. If he could find a way to block VEGF, Dr. Ferrara surmised, perhaps he could in turn impede tumor growth.

By the time EntreMed's drugs were falling short, Genentech had finally found its VEGF blocker. The company quickly scaled up the research and was soon testing the drug, which it called Avastin (bevacizumab), against all sorts of cancers in humans. In June 2003, the company reported its first success: Avastin prolonged median survival in advanced colon cancer patients from about 16 months to slightly more than 20 months when compared with standard chemotherapy alone. In February 2004, the FDA approved Avastin for the treatment of metastatic colorectal cancer in combination with standard chemotherapy.

Avastin was the first official anti-angiogenesis drug—and, Genentech hoped, not the last. As of 2009, the company was testing Avastin in more than 450 clinical trials, against more than 30 different kinds of cancer. A great number of these have failed to show results, but there have been certain successes. In addition to late-stage colon cancer, Avastin has been approved by the FDA for use against metastatic breast cancer, and an aggressive form of brain cancer known as glioblastoma, and the most common kind of lung cancer.

This hit-and-miss record makes Avastin a drug that suits the times. On the one hand, it's not the cure-all for cancer that Dr. Folkman's theory of anti-angiogenesis seemed to promise. The theory may have been vindicated, but the particulars of the biology have proven to be wilier than expected. On the other hand, Avastin has been shown to have *specific* benefits against *specific* cancers in *specific* stages.

The challenge for physicians and patients alike, then, is to appreciate those specifics and use the drug strategically. This is especially important since the drug is so expensive: Annual costs can easily soar to $100,000, and patients can be on the hook for 20 percent or more of that. What's more, it's important to realize what it means when we say that Avastin "works." Genentech's best results have shown extensions of between 2 and 4 months of life on average. That was sufficient for FDA approval, and those few months will be blessed days for cancer patients (of course, some patients will respond better to the drug and survive much longer than that average, while others who don't respond will have a shorter survival time). But it's important for a patient to be fully aware of that limited effect. Avastin is an extender, not a cure, and even then it's been shown to work in only the most precise circumstances.

Take lung cancer, for example. The FDA didn't approve the drug for treating lung cancer, broadly speaking. The approval stipulated that the drug should be used in combination with two chemotherapy drugs in patients with "unresectable, locally advanced, recurrent or metastatic non-squamous non-small cell lung carcinoma." There's a great deal of precision in that approval. And even for those patients, the clinical trial found that Avastin extended the average survival time by only 2 months, from 10.3 months to 12.3 months. Are 2 months worth $100,000? How about $200,000? It's a difficult question to answer, and the verdict depends largely on who's answering and who's paying.

Or consider colon cancer. Again, the FDA set down precise parameters for using Avastin: It should be used along with chemotherapy in patients with advanced colorectal cancer or for those who have already undergone treatment. In other words, for colon cancer patients this is a drug of last resort. Despite its efforts and hundreds of expensive trials, Genentech has had a hard time making it more than that. In early 2009 the company announced that a study of Avastin as an early stage treatment for colon cancer had failed to pan out, thwarting the company's hopes for a broader market.

Of course, to some extent that broader market will come to Avastin anyway, despite the FDA's circumspect approvals. The FDA allows physicians to prescribe approved drugs for any condition at their discretion. These so-called "off label" uses happen all the time, so inevitably, there will be early stage colon cancer patients out there who demand and receive Avastin, even though it hasn't been shown to have any effect on these cancers. Similarly, Avastin is surely being used for early breast cancers and other cancers by patients who are grasping for anything that might help.

The limited effects of Avastin also make clear how clinical trials can so often be sirens' songs of false hope. Cancer patients are particularly vulnerable to this, since they're often searching for one last shot at survival. But in truth, most drugs don't work, and the odds that an experimental treatment will work better than anything already out there are, statistically speaking, slim to none.

It's also important to recognize that phase I trials aren't designed to test for effectiveness. By definition, a phase I trial tests for *toxicity*—how dangerous the drug is in various amounts—not whether or how well it works. That means dosages are typically limited to a fraction of what's hypothesized to be an effective dose. So even if the drug *does work,* it's unlikely that the trial subject is getting enough for it to have any effect.

In practice, though, patients often misunderstand the purpose of a phase I trial. Many people, especially those with cancer, think getting into a clinical trial is a last shot at survival. A 2006 study showed that fewer than half of patients enrolled in cancer research understood the purpose of a phase I trial, with many believing they would benefit from the trial. The pharmaceutical industry needs to do a much better job of making it clear to these patients that they have little to gain from a phase I study. Their participation should clearly stem from the hope that it may benefit others down the road, not that they themselves actually stand a chance of benefiting.

In 2008, the *New York Times* ran another front-page story on anti-angiogenesis drugs, this one as part of a series entitled The Evidence Gap. The story meticulously poked holes in the allure of Avastin, noting that its expense, limited effectiveness, and broad off-label usage make it of dubious benefit for most patients and nothing more than a false hope for many. On the byline: Gina Kolata, the same reporter whose story about Dr. Folkman had caused such a furor a decade earlier.

JUDAH FOLKMAN DIED IN JANUARY 2008. His obituaries properly hailed him as a man of great courage, someone willing to be considered wrong for years. Indeed, part of the lesson of Dr. Folkman's work is that a good idea shouldn't be left on the shelf, that even an apparently foolish observation can turn out to be the best science. His willingness to challenge the orthodoxy of chemotherapy and suggest that there are other ways to approach the problem of cancer was, for decades, considered sheer lunacy. But when vindication finally came, Dr. Folkman didn't gloat. He kept working. He kept researching the problem.

The pharmaceutical industry, on the other hand, has taken a very narrow road toward its billion-dollar business model. Once a drug is approved, research largely stops (Genentech's 450 Avastin trials are an exception). The marginal efficacy rates of most drugs are considered acceptable, and rarely is an effort made to improve those numbers by narrowing the population pool taking the drug (after all, if a drug that's 50 percent effective is taken only by those for whom it works, well, that would be half as many people buying the drug).

When follow-up research is conducted, though, it can be remarkably revealing and informative. ALLHAT and STAR*D both demonstrated that there's more to learn about how drugs work in individuals. Both of these studies were unprecedented in scale and ambition. And they were funded by the government (not drug companies) and sought to encompass the reality of how we use pharmaceuticals instead of taking place within the false sterility of a clinical trial. And both started in the mid-1990s.

It's high time, then, for another era of similar research that goes still a step further. Matching drugs to individuals doesn't require following a fad like pharmacogenomics, and it's hardly dependent on the recalcitrant drug companies. A wealth of knowledge has been cast aside in the study of drugs, the product of good research that, given a second look, could pinpoint new molecules that might help people. This approach—drug rescue, as it's called in the industry—shouldn't be left to the industry.

In the interests of true openness, the owners of this fallow research, this unexploited data, should be compelled to contribute it to a collective repository that could be exploited by anybody—number crunchers, entrepreneurs, even patients. Personalized medicine shouldn't have to wait for the next billion-dollar breakthrough.

9

On the Horns of a Dilemma

Making Smarter Decisions about Treating Disease

I.

KOLYA KIRIENKO WAS 17 when he was diagnosed with Crohn's disease. In retrospect, he had known something was wrong for years, but he wasn't inclined to admit it. An especially driven teenager, Kolya was an outstanding student at a San Diego military academy and had been selected to join the prestigious Air Force Academy. "I had it all planned," he says a decade later. "I was going to be a pilot and serve for 30 years. I was going to be a lifer, then maybe join an airline. I was ready. But all of that unraveled with the diagnosis."

Crohn's is an enigmatic disease. It's difficult to diagnose, and its signs and symptoms are sometimes wrongly dismissed as psychosomatic in origin (it's often mistaken for anorexia nervosa, among other conditions). Long thought to be an autoimmune disorder, Crohn's is more accurately described as an acute inflammatory process. It can affect the entire gastrointestinal tract, from the mouth to the anus. The condition is painful, but even worse is that the inflammation makes it difficult to digest food, resulting in frequent gastrointestinal distress and persistent nutritional deficiencies. In other words, the body refuses to do its job;

rather than processing the food you eat, your intestines perceive it as a threat and reject it in any number of ways. If the inflammation is severe enough, it can turn stretches of the intestines into scar tissue, resulting in blockages that restrict food from making its way through the body. Though there is no cure, there are treatments. But for those with the condition, it can be devastatingly disruptive to ordinary life—as Kolya learned when he read that his condition disqualified him from entering the US Air Force. His life plan had hit a brick wall.

It took Kolya a while to comprehend his new reality, distracted as he was by the months he spent in the hospital as doctors struggled to treat his condition. "Everybody says Crohn's isn't that serious; you take prednisone [an immunosuppressant corticosteroid] and have some belly pain, but you're basically fine," he recalls. "My experience was nothing like that. I didn't respond to anything they gave me. I was in extreme pain and couldn't eat. I was fed through an IV for 6 months." Finally, in August 1999, he opted for surgery to remove the scar tissue obstructing his intestine.

At first it seemed that he was cured. Seventeen days after his surgery, Kolya climbed Half Dome in Yosemite National Park, toasting the achievement by eating a turkey sandwich at the top. "I'd dreamt of that sandwich for months," he recalls. But within a few months, the pain started to come back, along with the swollen belly that is symptomatic of a bowel obstruction. And soon he was back in the operating room for another surgery.

Today, Kolya is a tall, gangly 28-year-old with a wispy blond goatee. He is shy but friendly, with an engaging smile. Though Crohn's is, as he says, "an invisible chronic illness," his pale complexion and taciturn bearing testify to the decade he's spent quietly struggling with the disease. Since he was diagnosed, Kolya has had five surgeries to remove blocked sections of scarred sections of blocked intestine; he's also had kidney surgery, a consequence of years of undiagnosed illness. Along the way, he has taken a drugstore's worth of medications. Some block the body's inflammatory response. Others treat the side effects caused by these medications (necessary because the immune system is no longer fighting other battles). He also requires periodic infusions of vitamin B_{12}, iron, and other nutritional boosters to compensate for constant anemia. And he tops it all off with significant doses of pain medication. Each of these comes with its own strict timetable, possible side effects, and potential interactions. And each one requires a painstaking process of consideration, evaluation, and monitoring to ensure that the risks are outweighed by the rewards.

Over the past 10 years, Kolya has developed an expert, firsthand knowledge of the medical system and the demands it makes on individuals. He's learned that a case like his generates a huge volume of records that require almost constant management. "I've been discharged from a hospital 27 times. Over the course of 10 years, I've had so many providers that my case is very siloed among hospitals," he says, referring to how every institution keeps separate files. He's learned that major choices about treatment can happen in an instant. "You meet with your doctor and you've got 15 minutes to make these intense decisions, like which drug will I take, a drug that costs $80,000 a year. With 15 minutes!"

He's learned that he alone is the ultimate steward of his own health; indeed, at times, he has made choices that were against the recommendations of his doctors. "I've asked for surgeries when they didn't want to, and it was the right decision. I have to ask for an iron infusion to fight my anemia. They'll give it to me when I ask, but no one was owning my case. Except me."

Tracking all this is taxing, but thankfully, it's something that Kolya is well suited to. He's at home with a computer, working on spreadsheets that chart his dosages and side effects. But he realizes that most people aren't so lucky.

The severity of their situations notwithstanding, pretty much everyone who crosses paths with modern medicine will find that gathering and processing the available information can be the biggest challenge of being a patient. Decisions are many, science is scarce, and the risks are always high. Treating a disease is complicated, and "there are no standards for making these decisions," Kolya says. "And that's made worse by the fact that people may be in a reduced cognitive state because they're sick. We all need a better way to manage our health."

THIS BOOK STARTED with the premise that preventive measures are our best shot at having long and healthy lives. But there's no ignoring the fact that, eventually, we will all get sick. And when a serious disease does strike, our choices and their consequences only become more fraught. Because the stakes are so high, it's a point when many of us may prefer to stop trying to direct our own health care. Let the doctors take over, we say, let the insurance company decide what constitutes effective care, let me get back to controlling what I can control: My bank account. My relationships. But not, alas, my health.

But the fact is, even for physicians, treatment is a confused and muddled art. Despite the emphasis in medicine on diagnosis and treatment, the act of prognosis—of estimating what a patient's potential outcomes are—is poorly taught in medical schools. Too often, physicians operate on gut instinct rather than scientific evidence. And when they do turn to evidence, there's no guarantee they'll correctly interpret it: In a classic 1982 study of physician reasoning, the mathematician and physician David Eddy, MD, PhD, asked 100 doctors to interpret a probability that a patient has breast cancer based on a positive mammogram. Nearly all the physicians mistakenly predicted that the patient was 75 percent likely to have breast cancer—even though the correct answer, given the vagaries of false positives, was about 10 times less, actually about 7 percent. Dr. Eddy's study did, it should be mentioned, inaugurate the era of what's known as "evidence-based medicine," and the years since have seen medical education placing a marked emphasis on statistical inference and reasoning.

Still, even when a doctor does turn to actual science rather than a hunch and does correctly interpret the evidence for a prognosis, he's not actually talking about you. More correctly, he's talking about what happened to a group of people back in some research study and then applying that general result to your specific situation. When a study shows that people with, say, a particular form of cancer at a particular stage have 6 months of expected life left at the time of diagnosis, that 6 months is an *average,* based on what happened in the larger population.

Now, you, well, you're unlikely to reach 6 months and then just drop dead. You will live either less time than that or more than that—probably just a little less or more, but maybe a lot. Sure, somewhere there is an objective truth, but because it exists in the future, you're left with a statistical estimate. Since we typically cannot, as Vesalius would have, crack you open and produce certainty, your doctor is left with an abstraction based on previous research. This is known as the expectation principle, and it frequently trips up patients and physicians alike. A textbook for physicians underscores the logical problem in discussing how to share information about a patient's prognosis: "Because we do not know in advance, *at the time of the decision*, whether a particular patient will be one of the lucky ones or one of the unlucky ones, each patient is in an identical state of uncertainty and faces the same expected, or average, loss." But that abstract average is unlikely to precisely correspond to the actual fate of any one patient.

In a broader sense, all treatment decisions are statistical estimates, best guesses that substitute for the unknowable objective truth that looms out there. You will or you won't get cancer (there's no such thing as getting 40 percent of a cancer), a drug will work or it won't (as discussed in Chapter 8, fifty-fifty odds is considered good), you will die of this disease or you won't. But since we cannot know these things for certain, we must estimate, interrogating the odds with the best tools and formulas at our disposal. These are data in their rawest form. They say a lot, but they say almost nothing specifically about you.

This is the great hazard inherent in making decisions about medical treatments: We must confront the momentous uncertainties that life inextricably contains. Uncertainty has been present throughout this book; it is at the root, if you will, of every Decision Tree we might confront, from those dealing with genetic risks to screening tests to drug choices. Uncertainty looms in every health choice we make, just as it factors into all aspects of life. There is no sure thing, and just as the courses of our lives, in general, are bowed and bent by unexpected events, so too does our health, in particular, course along uncertain trajectories. We can try to predict where things may go, we can try to prevent the worst from happening, we can try to extend the good and minimize the bad.

But every action and every decision is part of a process beset by things we do not and often cannot know.

Not that uncertainty is always a bad thing. In many ways, uncertainty is our ally, especially in matters of health. Another way to think of uncertainty, after all, is hope. The chance that something may turn out better than expected, that even a small probability of success will prevail, is something that we cling to, especially when our straits turn dire. In another sense, uncertainty is the very essence of choice, affirming that we are individuals imbued with the human right of autonomy. Not all of these choices will turn out for the best (that is the trade-off of choice: we have to live with the consequences). But the fact that we have options, that we have some input in dictating the courses of our lives, this is the very essence of humanity. Call it free will or whatever you like, but it's there thanks to the uncertainty manifest in life itself.

Of course, this is indulgent philosophizing when the uncertainty before you is a matter of life and death, or close to it, like that faced by Kolya Kirienko. A decade into the 21st century, we expect much of medicine—and sometimes, a candid physician may confess, we expect too much. For medicine is the opportunistic flushing out of uncertainty, bit by bit, and though we know a lot, there is a great deal that is still unknown.

In an academic sense, uncertainty is simply the stuff of science. As a process of discovery, the purpose of science is to confront uncertainty with precise questions, methods, and purpose, in the hope of illuminating what was previously obscure. But where in most sciences this process is an acceptable abstraction (establishing whether string theory is right or wrong isn't really going to change anybody's life either way), there's less tolerance for the process in medical science. In fact, a century of steady advancements in medicine has created the popular presumption that most of the answers are already known, that for most conditions the right treatment sits out there someplace on the shelf. For most of us, it's only when we personally reckon with disease that we confront the vast imperfections of medicine. The foggy presence of uncertainty becomes manifestly obvious when the question of what to do is plunked before us.

Uncertainty is especially vexing because we, as humans, can't help but turn life into a story, a narrative imbued with meaning and purpose. Uncertainty exposes this habit as a ruse. The brutal biological fact is that, despite whatever meaning we may find in it, life is largely ruled by random chance. We are animals, after all, subject to the same vagaries of disease and accident that apes and antelopes are. Our conscious desire for control imposes order upon this randomness.

Numerous psychological experiments have established that, even in situations where we have no control—lotteries, casino gambling, spectator sports—we behave as if we do have control. We *try* to wield control, even when it's impossible to do so. This goes back to Dr. Michael Marmot's work in the Whitehall studies—being able to control our destinies is everything. This is a side effect of our self-conscious natures, which in so many other regards give us pleasure and joy. Self-consciousness, after all, allows us to feel love and pride and empathy. But it also compels us to search for order where there is none, to assume truth where there is only uncertainty. It is, as this chapter will explore further, the classic conflict between rationality and emotion. And in a situation where a disease has struck, the two get all entwined. Our emotional sides appeal to the rationality of medicine for some objective answer, though there is often no one answer to be had.

So much for the philosophy. Here's why I belabor the point: The appeal of a Decision Tree, given our desire for control and meaning, is that it can help us to recognize what, in fact, we *do* have control over and help us to exercise that control to our best advantage. A Decision Tree framework can acknowledge uncertainty while helping us to focus on what we do know and which levers we can adjust.

It's worth reminding ourselves, now, of just what a "good decision" actually means in medicine. First and foremost, it means a decision that leads to a better outcome. We want to choose the treatment that either cures us or allows us to manage disease in a way that lets us make the most of our lives. But a good decision can also mean the best *possible* decision, one that is carefully considered, draws on all relevant information (and avoids irrelevant information), and is consistent with how we want to live our lives. It is in this latter sense that this chapter will use the term.

When our health has gone off course and we are beset by disease, we need to make the smartest, best-informed decisions possible. We need to engage with uncertainty and elevate it, flush it out and confront it, in order to see our way more clearly to what our prognosis truly is and what our options truly are. After all, a century ago there was likely *less* uncertainty about matters of health: Then, we were healthy until we weren't. When disease struck, there wasn't much that could be done about it; maybe there were a few drugs that might hurt as much as they could help, and the field of surgery was one step removed from the barbershop. The odds were much worse, but the truth was a lot more apparent.

In contrast, the opportunity we have today is to make things *more complicated,* thus expanding our options. We want to bring more information into the equation in order to reduce uncertainty wherever it may be. The trick is—and this is no small thing—to find a way to parse this surfeit of information without being overwhelmed, without throwing up our hands and leaving our fate to the judgment of our physicians alone. After all, for all their skills and smarts, physicians are often less equipped to weigh what constitutes the best options and outcomes than the patients themselves are. When making a treatment decision, in other words, is precisely when we need a Decision Tree the most: when it will allow us to weigh the options and the odds, assess the implications and the outcomes, consult the experts and the evidence, and make the choice that suits us best.

OF ALL THE TRICKS, techniques, and strategies for making better decisions, few have improved upon the one suggested by Ben Franklin back in 1772. In writing to a friend, he offered a method for parsing information and coming to a sound judgment:

> My way is to divide half a sheet of paper by a line into two columns; writing over the one *Pro,* and over the other *Con.* Then during three or four days' consideration I put down

under the different heads short hints of the different motives that at different times occur to me, *for* or *against* the measure. When I have thus got them all together in one view, I endeavour to estimate their respective weights; and where I find two (one on each side) that seem equal, I strike them both out. If I find a reason *pro* equal to some two reasons *con*, I strike out the three. If I judge some two reasons *con* equal to some three reasons *pro*, I strike out the five; and thus proceeding I find at length where the balance lies; and if after a day or two of farther consideration nothing new that is of importance occurs on either side, I come to a determination accordingly. And though the weight of reasons cannot be taken with the precision of algebraic quantities, yet when each is thus considered separately and comparatively, and the whole lies before me, I think I can judge better, and am less liable to make a rash step; and in fact I have found great advantage from this kind of equation in what may be called *moral* or *prudential algebra*.

The central element in Franklin's prudential algebra is a list of pros and cons—but it's much more than just that. Franklin sketched out a procedure for thinking through a problem and evaluating evidence and then for *reevaluating* a problem when new information presents itself. It is a fluid, flexible strategy that leaves the decision maker in control and requires him or her to engage with all the available relevant information while ignoring the irrelevant. Sketched out as a Decision Tree, Franklin's method looks like the chart on the next page.

The wisdom of Franklin's approach is that it takes advantage of the way we're already inclined to think something through. It just has us pause and do it with a little more consideration, without rushing to judgment. It doesn't require us to become experts in statistics or absorb years of medical research (unrealistic tasks for the best of us). It just asks us to consider what we do know, weigh the risks against the rewards, and use our own faculties for reason. It asks us to look before we leap.

For an example of Franklin's algebra in action, consider the example

Ben Franklin's Decision Tree Model

The founding father's "prudential algebra" neatly translates into a model Decision Tree for weighing facts and making a wise choice.

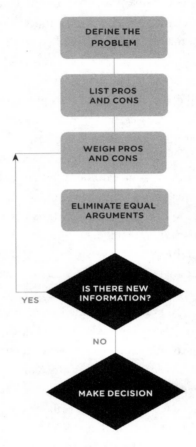

of a group of men with prostate cancer who have been working with Dean Ornish, MD, on behavioral treatments for the disease. Every month, the group gathers in Dr. Ornish's office in Sausalito, California, to discuss their disease status; their progress in sticking with Dr. Ornish's low-fat, vegetarian diet and exercise program; and their lives in general. It's an uncommon approach, particularly for men who've already been diagnosed with cancer. "When I was diagnosed, I was told by my urologists that I had two choices," group member Dennis Simkin said. "Radiation or surgery. There wasn't a lot of talk about anything else. But then

I heard about this group and realized there was a third option, that there were behaviors that might reduce the chances that this cancer would kill us, without surgery or radiation. This idea that there was a third choice, another path, was completely unexpected."

Dr. Ornish has had particular success with this third path. A 3-month study of 30 patients with low-grade prostate cancer found that after making intensive lifestyle modifications—following a low-fat, vegetarian diet coupled with exercise, meditation, and weekly group meetings—the men's average PSA level dropped slightly while their free PSA (a positive measure of prostate health) climbed. And what's more, measures of stress, weight, and blood pressure had all improved. And it goes further still: The study found significant improvements on a genetic level, both in terms of gene expression and on what's called the telomeres of the chromosomes—the ends of the strands in our DNA that are protective of long life.

I should quickly add that this path isn't for everyone. Many men diagnosed with prostate cancer will still prefer to go the route of radiation or surgery. Others might consider something like the customized information delivered by Soar BioDynamics, discussed in Chapter 6. But that's not the point. The takeaway is this: Dennis Simkin thought there were only two options, both of them potentially destructive to his life. But then he discovered that in fact there were more choices, a discovery that would turn out to add something to his life. His Decision Tree offered him choices that he hadn't known existed. He just had to learn where to look.

Not all treatment decisions are as simple as putting one more option on the table. They require balancing handfuls of options with dozens of implications and weighing untold unknowns. In the past decade, the science of medical decision making has come into its own, developing a great many intriguing strategies to help improve choices by physicians and patients alike. But the volume of information has become a problem in itself, a great and constant distraction that may inhibit us in making the right calls. The rest of this chapter will explore these opportunities and obstacles, and look at how we may be able to make better decisions—and why some choices will always be poor bets.

II.

WHEN MOST OF US FACE a medical question or decision, we start our search for information on the Internet. We Google. There's no shame in this; a bit of savvy searching can turn up the same research that our doctors consult. Resources like WebMD and MayoClinic.com are godsends, rich in clear, sound information that can leave us well versed and reassured. Primary research material is available from MEDLINE at PubMed (www.pubmed.gov), where anybody can read abstracts from medical research and download many complete papers, free of charge. But not every search leads us to clarity; there is plenty of garbage on the Web, and following a link or two can lead us down some decidedly dubious paths.

For doctors, the Internet has been a mixed blessing. For time-pressed physicians, it relieves some of the burden of making explanations and providing background. But it has also led to a class of patients some physicians dismiss as "Googlers," people who are either misinformed or overdemanding and end up interfering with the courses of care their doctors would have them follow.

This isn't an idle problem. The first challenge in making good decisions is finding good information. Bad information isn't just worthless, it can be destructive. "Garbage in, garbage out," as they say in computer science, meaning that any process that starts with bad data will result in only bad conclusions. And given that the Internet contains more than its share of garbage, it's not hard to imagine that it can have some negative effects. The question is, does it help or hurt? Can people separate the good from the bad?

This was the question that Eric Horvitz decided to answer. An expert in artificial intelligence at Microsoft Research, Horvitz is a trained MD and has a PhD in computer science from Stanford. He talks in rapid-fire bursts, jumping from one topic to another as if he has to get his thought out before it disappears. Dr. Horvitz has spent most of the past 2 decades at least 10 years ahead of the curve, thinking about how computers can help patients and physicians make better diagnostic and treatment decisions. In the late 1980s at Stanford, Dr. Horvitz studied how artificial intelligence might be used to improve decision making. And in the mid-1990s, when the World Wide Web was just dawning, Dr. Horvitz developed an online guide for pregnancy and child care that used Bayesian logic models to help parents make simple decisions on coughs, runny noses, and bumps and bruises—the sort of thing that people are finally ready for today.

In 2007, Dr. Horvitz and a Microsoft colleague, Ryen White, PhD, wondered exactly how people engage with health information on the Internet. Do they click on the garbage and study it just as hard as the good stuff? Or do they somehow discern the quality from the crap and emerge better informed?

Dr. Horvitz didn't want to know what people *said* they did online; questionnaires about Internet use are notoriously incomplete and imprecise. He wanted to know what they *really* did. He wanted to follow people and watch them. And since he and Dr. White worked at Microsoft, they realized they actually had a way to find out. Dr. Horvitz and Dr. White collected 11 months of user logs, containing millions of searches from Microsoft's MSN search engine and MSN Health and Fitness, a popular online health resource. Users had consented to allow their searches to be used for research, and details that could identify the users were stripped out to make the data anonymous. But anyway, finding what individuals did wasn't the point—they wanted to see what *thousands* of people did.

They started with searches for 12 common symptoms—headache, chest pain, muscle twitches, rash, fatigue, fever, and so on—and looked at which Web sites people ended up on. In reality, these symptoms are so common that they're almost always either benign or due to something mild. A headache, for instance, is usually a symptom of something like caffeine withdrawal. Muscle twitches happen to most people now and again, and they go away with rest and time. But the Web wasn't leading people to these conclusions. Quite the contrary: The Web was leading people to think the worst. People searching for "headache" ended up spending just as much time reading about brain tumors—which are exceptionally rare, happening in perhaps 1 in 16,000 Americans—as caffeine withdrawal. People with muscle twitches spent half their time reading about amyotrophic lateral sclerosis, or Lou Gehrig's disease, even though the average American's chance of developing it is 1 in 800.

What's more, Dr. Horvitz and Dr. White found that once people started thinking the worst, they couldn't stop. They would return to the Web to research worst-case scenarios like brain tumors again and again. And months after their initial searches, they would interrupt other searches and return to searching "brain tumor." They couldn't get the worst-case scenarios out of their heads. Dr. Horvitz calls this phenomenon "cyberchondria," a particular, Internet-induced form of hypochondria that can afflict even the most sophisticated Web users.

The problem, Dr. Horvitz says, is that the Web just isn't suited for the sort of medical decision making that people want to use it for. "When you're deciding between a Sony camera and a Canon, the Web is great. When there are clear trade-offs in outcomes, people say the Web works." These are what are called evaluative questions, queries that seek answers involving values and worth. But, Dr. Horvitz explained, people searching for health information are often asking inferential questions, those that require some interpretation and outside knowledge. And that just doesn't compute. "The Web doesn't understand things like probabilities and associations. The Web has no probability information. There's no base rate on the Internet.

"This isn't to say people shouldn't be using the Web," Dr. Horvitz continues. "They will be using the Web. But we need to make a better Web. When somebody's using the Web to make diagnosis or treatment decisions, it should recognize that and guide them toward credible models for prediction and advice."

Dr. Horvitz and his team at Microsoft Research are working on creating such systems that can pull Internet users toward good information, rather than sending them toward the dubious and doubtful. (Microsoft's Bing search engine reflects some of this thinking by recognizing many common medical searches and matching them with tailored results.) But more broadly, his research demonstrates that when we seek medical advice, as opposed to advice on buying a DVD player or a dishwasher, we're especially vulnerable to poor or inappropriate or excessive information. That can lead to unnecessary worry, ill-founded self-treatments, and any number of bad decisions.

It's the same sort of problem that was discussed in Chapter 4: The problem isn't a lack of information, it's a lack of a way to process it. The more we understand why that is—why we're likely to go astray just when we shouldn't—the more we can stop treating our case of sniffles like it's the swine flu.

A POP QUIZ: Say you have a serious disease, one that needs to be treated with a drug. If you don't receive treatment, your risk of dying over the next year is 10 percent. There are two medications available, Drug A and Drug B. They cost the same, and neither has significant side effects. But you can take only one.

If you take Drug A, it will decrease your risk of dying by 80 percent over the next year.

If 100 people with the disease take Drug B, eight deaths will be prevented over the next year.

Which do you take?

In a survey of about 500 patients, 57 percent chose Drug A, and just 15 percent chose Drug B (another 15 percent were indifferent). The truth is, of course, that the effects are exactly the same. Since there's only a 10 percent risk of dying, the fact that Drug B saved eight lives means that it worked in 80 percent of cases—the same outcome as with Drug A. The difference is only in how the two outcomes are presented. Drug A is presented as a relative risk, the risk compared to other risks. Drug B, on the other hand, is presented as an absolute risk, in this case the overall risk of death. The benefit of relative risk is that it is personalized and connects an individual to his or her own choices. The problem with relative risk is that it is often misleading, both in terms of one's risk for disease and in terms of the hope offered by a certain treatment.

Now consider this survey, given to about 250 physicians and patients. They were asked this question:

Please imagine that you are a patient with a very serious medical condition. Your physician tells you that there are two treatments available for your condition, treatments A and B. Your physician's opinion is that you should be treated, because the consequences of non-treatment are infinitely worse than treatment. Your physician would like to know your preferences for the treatments to help him/her decide which of the two treatments should be used in your particular case. I will be asking you which of the treatments you would choose if you were the patient.

The respondents were then shown one of two tables of survival rates, as follows:

Summary Data at Six Discrete Time Points

| | Number of Patients out of 100 | |
	Treatment A	Treatment B
After 1 month	90 alive; 10 dead	100 alive; 0 dead
After 1 year	68 alive; 32 dead	77 alive; 23 dead
After 2 years	51 alive; 49 dead	48 alive; 52 dead
After 3 years	40 alive; 60 dead	28 alive; 72 dead
After 4 years	35 alive; 65 dead	23 alive; 77 dead
After 5 years	34 alive; 66 dead	22 alive; 78 dead

Summary Data at Three Discrete Time Points

| | Number of Patients out of 100 | |
	Treatment A	Treatment B
After 1 month	90 alive; 10 dead	100 alive; 0 dead
After 1 year	68 alive; 32 dead	77 alive; 23 dead
After 5 years	34 alive; 66 dead	22 alive; 78 dead

These are, of course, the same survival rates over 5 years, but Table 1 shows survival at six points while Table 2 shows just three points. A small difference, but a dramatic one: People shown Table 2 were evenly split, fifty-fifty, between the treatments, while those shown the more detailed Table 1 greatly preferred Treatment A, 84 percent to 16 percent.

The difference, it seems, was that Table 2 emphasized mortality, so the decision became a toss-up because neither treatment seems especially good. But the detail in Table 1 frames the treatments in a more positive light; the choice became a matter of maximizing survival rather than minimizing death—and in that circumstance, Treatment A seems overwhelmingly superior.

These examples illustrate how vulnerable we are to the ways that medical information is presented, and how apparently slight changes in description or emphasis can lead us to radically different conclusions. Such considerations—what researchers call framing—are just one factor in helping people make sound medical decisions.

The two-tables example also illustrates how we're prone to misreading the circumstances when the decision has a long-term horizon. Most humans, behavioral economists have found, have something called a discount rate—an innate tendency to discount long-term gains in favor of short-term benefits. This discount varies from person to person; studies have found that people with more education have longer discount rates than those with less (a correlation that seems related to the link between more education and better health in general).

And even when we do understand the statistics we're given, well, we're prone to distorting what they say in some very telling ways. By and large, people are also prone to thinking they have better chances than they do. Numerous psychological studies have shown that, when asked to compare themselves with others, patients routinely say that they are doing better than the average patient would, and that their chances of successful treatment or survival are better than the odds would suggest. In other words, even when the odds of successful treatment are slim, say a 10 percent chance, people tend to categorize themselves among those few for whom things will work out. We assume we're going to be in that 10 percent of the lucky ones.

Psychologists call this the Lake Wobegon effect, playing off humorist Garrison Keillor's yarns about the town where everybody is above average. (There may be a benefit to such optimism, unrealistic though it may be: Still other studies have shown that thinking positively can become a self-fulfilling prophecy, especially in cases that involve physical therapy or similar intensive, rigorous treatment.)

All of which is to say: When it comes to understanding the facts, assessing our options, and making good decisions about our health, we humans can be very slippery, and frequently misguided, creatures. The cumulative lesson of cyberchondria, the Lake Wobegon effect, and other examples of poor decision making is this: When individuals are confronted with a medical situation, we are awfully likely to choose poorly, left to our own devices. But there's a silver lining: Knowing our inherent limitations may be the secret to getting us to choose wisely next time.

IN THE 1980S, VALERIE REYNA, PHD, was a freshly minted psychologist studying how people make decisions. At the time, the topic had been paid little attention. The presumption then (as it still often is today) was that getting people to make better decisions was simply a matter of giving them more information. The better informed people are, the better equipped they should be to make good decisions.

But the data didn't bear that out. In fact, several studies seemed to show that the amount somebody knew about a problem, in terms of facts and figures, had pretty much no bearing on the value of their subsequent decisions. The quality of people's memories had nothing to do with the quality of their reasoning, says Dr. Reyna, who today is a professor of human development and psychology and a codirector of the Center for Behavioral Economics and Decision Research at Cornell University in Ithaca, New York.

Instead, what seemed to be happening was that people were acting on the basis of how well they grasped the gist of a problem, the bottom-line meaning rather than the particulars. That meaning, not surprisingly, is heavily influenced by all the other stuff the decision maker brings to the table—experiences, biases, and so forth. In other words, "expertise" didn't matter nearly as much as having an intuitive understanding of a problem and what their goals were.

Dr. Reyna called her observation "fuzzy trace theory" in an attempt to describe the roundabout and fuzzy way most decisions are reached. As the name suggests, fuzzy trace theory is just a theory; it's an interpretation of how our minds work, an attempt to describe the way we make decisions so that advice might be given to guide us toward better decisions. And it could be wrong. The chemistry of our brains could work in an entirely different way that fuzzy trace theory fails to recognize. But increasingly, the theory has found supporters in the psychological and medical communities because it *feels* right; it seems to fit the evidence. It explains both the reason why throwing more information at a decision doesn't improve outcomes and also the reason some people make good decisions even when they aren't schooled in the specifics. Improving our memories, in other words, doesn't improve our ability to reason.

The practical implications of Dr. Reyna's theory are several. Fuzzy trace theory would argue for information to be presented in terms of relative risks, where we get closest to our own outcomes, rather than absolute risks, which are technically accurate but abstract and difficult to understand in personal terms. It would encourage the use of Venn diagrams and bar charts rather than tables and raw data so we can better process the gist of the information and not be distracted by specific numbers. And it would guide medical providers to be mindful and consider the language they use to present treatment options to patients so the framing of information doesn't play on our prejudices and distort our judgments (when the short-term discomfort of a treatment is emphasized over its long-term benefits, for instance, patients may choose not to undergo treatments that would in fact meet their goals of living longer lives). It would insist that it's more important to know that there's *some* risk to a procedure rather than to memorize the specific percentage of risk. "If you know how people make decisions," Dr. Reyna says, "then you can help them make better decisions."

It's important to note that fuzzy trace theory applies to the judgment of patients and physicians alike. Doctors are just as likely as patients to go on gut instinct; indeed, given their time demands and training, they're perhaps *more* likely to go by their guts. For example, fuzzy trace theory explains why all those doctors surveyed by Dr. Eddy thought that the patient's actual risk of breast cancer was 75 percent and not 7 percent. They were going by their guts and making judgment calls. But they called it wrong.

As Jerome Groopman, MD, explored in his important book *How*

Doctors Think, most physicians make decisions using heuristics, or rules of thumb. Heuristics are the holy sacraments of medicine, the dogmas that have been passed along from doctor to doctor, drilled into them in medical school and internships until they've become instincts. But these heuristics are notoriously dodgy; they may or may not be supported by evidence. For instance, an emergency room physician might get used to seeing one or two coronary patients come through the ER a day. Therefore, on a day that brings in no coronary patients, this doctor can easily be predisposed to too quickly diagnosing a heart attack when a patient with vague symptoms does come in (this heuristic is known as the gambler's fallacy). As a 2008 paper in the journal *Medical Decision Making* put it, "We can hold no illusions that clinicians ordinarily make perfectly rational decisions. They do not. Like other humans, [physicians] apply cognitive heuristics that simplify but also distort the decision maker's appraisal of information."

At first glance, fuzzy trace theory seems like bad news for a Decision Tree approach. If physician and patient alike are prone to choosing poorly, left to our own devices, what's to become of us? If we're not good at processing information, then what good are collecting and tracking our personal data, trying to make better-informed behavior changes, and detecting problems early if we're going to fall back on our habits and hunches anyway?

But that's not exactly what fuzzy trace theory is telling us. In fact, fuzzy trace theory is telling us that if there is anything to be learned about our health, if there is any information to bring to our situation, we'd better understand it—*really* understand it—and appreciate what it means. Otherwise, it's just noise. Think of it this way: Fuzzy trace theory offers a way to acknowledge what we're good at and what we're not. But if we know we're predisposed to favoring intuition over statistics, maybe we can game our own system so that, in the end, we end up making the right decision.

The Decision Tree approach, after all, isn't about throwing information at a problem—there's already too much of that. It's about finding a way to parse information in a way that makes sense to us, in a way that aligns with our habits and beliefs. It's about finding tools and systems that can help us get to better decisions despite ourselves. When heuristics work, we should use them. But when they fail, we should find an alternative, a system for decision making that relies less on heuristics and more on a system like Ben Franklin's.

III.

ANNETTE O'CONNOR, PHD, HAS BEEN THINKING of ways to help individuals make better medical decisions for more than 20 years. A professor of nursing and epidemiology at the University of Ottawa in Ontario, she remembers the days when pregnancy tests used to be considered doctors-only information. "In the old days, everybody told you what to do: the priest, the doctor, the lawyer, the banker," she says. "They were the experts. That was the system. But that's not the best answer anymore. People need to be engaged right at the front."

Like Microsoft's Dr. Horvitz and Cornell's Dr. Reyna, Dr. O'Connor recognizes that the first challenge patients have is the tendency to collect too much information in what can be a self-defeating gesture. "When there are too many options, we become overwhelmed by information," she says. "There are too many things that we could do or could fix, and we become paralyzed." What Dr. O'Connor envisions is a portfolio of decision tools that creates a "friendly front end to the science." These tools would use statistical methods to give people facing medical decisions clear pictures of the alternatives before them. Rather than just splatting the statistics in front of them, a good tool would guide them through a process, so that "people could be much more engaged in the whole process, so that you can make a considered decision, weighing what matters to you." For example, if kidney disease invites a range of treatment options from dietary changes to drugs to dialysis to transplant, not every patient will be a candidate for every option. A tool that customizes options based on an individual profile is essential to helping people arrive at sound decisions rather than forcing them into misinformed choices.

As a first step toward this portfolio of tools, Dr. O'Connor's Ottawa

Health Research Institute (OHRI) has created an online inventory of more than 200 health situations, from acne and allergies, to gallstones and gastroesophageal reflux disease, to varicose veins, where computerized decision tools are available to help people understand their situations and make good calls. The OHRI has also posted a two-page paper tool that is basically an updated version of Franklin's prudential algebra—a generic form that stacks up pros and cons and gives people a clearer picture of what their options are and what decisions they feel are best. Designed simply and clearly, and able to winnow out irrelevant information whenever possible, these tools can have a remarkable impact on the quality of our decision making. (Physicians have their own decision tools available, such as the Adjuvant! program discussed in Chapter 8. They're proven to work better than heuristics alone; a 2005 review in *JAMA,* found that, of 40 computerized decision systems for physicians studied, about two-thirds made measurable improvements in physicians' patient-care performance.)

Do these tools actually help patients? Do they overcome our fuzzy thinking or confuse us all the more? To answer that question, Dr. O'Connor reviewed nearly 200 studies that assessed a specific decision tool. These tools helped patients face specific situations, from breast and colon cancers, to diabetes, to osteoporosis treatments. The cumulative answer divined from these 200 studies was that, yes, decision tools lead to better decisions, as demonstrated by all sorts of metrics. Fewer patients using decision aids reported feeling uncertain or unclear about their options, and more had made up their minds on a course of treatment after using a decision aid. What's more, patients using decision aids had better understandings of the risks and rewards of treatment (in other words, in the terms of fuzzy trace theory, they seemed to get the gist of the decision). Patients using decision aids seemed to get better care than those acting solely on their physician's guidance. And compellingly, patients chose less surgery when they understood their options. They preferred a behavioral or drug therapy over an invasive procedure 24 percent more often after consulting a decision aid. "They wanted to hold on to their organs," Dr. O'Connor explains. "There was less heart surgery, fewer prostatectomies, less removal of the uterus. It looked like with low information they said, 'Okay, fine, take it out.' But with a decision aid, more people realized that with a surgical solution come other risks for harm."

Decision tools can play an important role in managing chronic conditions as well. Take a condition like diabetes, which can be an especially demanding disease: It requires constant monitoring and regular treatment, all the patient's own responsibility, and it increases the risk of other conditions like heart disease. Researchers at the Mayo Clinic recently developed a tool called Statin Choice that helps patients with type 2 diabetes make the often confusing choice of whether or not to take statins to lower their risk of heart attacks. The tool is deceptively simple: The patient is handed a sheet of paper with four straightforward questions in big letters. "What is your risk of having a heart attack in the next 10 years?" is the first question, and below it is an estimate of the patient's risk, a calculation based on gender, age, how long he or she has had diabetes, whether he or she smokes, and a couple of blood test measurements. The patient is given a probable risk of a heart attack, followed by the caveat "Keep in mind that we do not know what will happen to you; if you were to have a heart attack we cannot tell when this will happen."

The second question is "What benefit can you expect from taking statins compared to not taking statins?" It makes the point with two sets of 100 faces. The first shows the risk without statins, with some smiley faces and some frowns, the number depending on the patient's risk of a heart attack. The second set shows what happens to 100 people taking statins, and in this set a handful of the frowns have turned into smiles. Those are the lives saved by statins. The third question asks them to acknowledge that there are some downsides and side effects (nausea, possible kidney damage), and the fourth question simply asks, "What do you want to do now?" and offers a few choices: take statins, don't Take statins, or talk it over with your doctor.

So what's the impact of such an ordinary set of questions? In a study Mayo researchers gave about 50 patients the personalized Statin Choice tool and another 50 a pamphlet about cholesterol and heart disease. After 3 months, the same number of patients in each group were

A Decision Tree for Statins

A simple decision tool like Statin Choice, developed by the Mayo Clinic, turns a few select pieces of personal data into a more precise calculation of the risk of heart attack. The tool leads users through a four-step process that helps them understand the benefits of statins as well as the risks—and helps them navigate to a decision. Here's what the options look like.

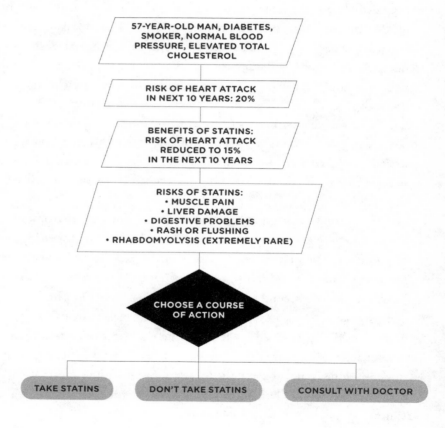

57-YEAR-OLD MAN, DIABETES, SMOKER, NORMAL BLOOD PRESSURE, ELEVATED TOTAL CHOLESTEROL

RISK OF HEART ATTACK IN NEXT 10 YEARS: 20%

BENEFITS OF STATINS: RISK OF HEART ATTACK REDUCED TO 15% IN THE NEXT 10 YEARS

RISKS OF STATINS:
• MUSCLE PAIN
• LIVER DAMAGE
• DIGESTIVE PROBLEMS
• RASH OR FLUSHING
• RHABDOMYOLYSIS (EXTREMELY RARE)

CHOOSE A COURSE OF ACTION

TAKE STATINS   DON'T TAKE STATINS   CONSULT WITH DOCTOR

taking statins. But their experience was otherwise quite different. The Statin Choice group showed a much better grasp of *why* they were taking statins, and they felt strongly that they understood their condition. What's more, the Statin Choice group missed fewer doses than those who'd been given the pamphlet—they were better at treating their disease.

Though there are fancier, more high-tech decision tools and strategies out there, the Statin Choice experiment makes two points quite clearly: First, a personalized description of treatment options seems far better than a generic presentation of facts. And second, breaking down the information into a series of linear steps is better than dumping the information on the patient all at once. By making the information about a particular person and letting them reach a decision step by step, Franklin style, the tool made the choice into something that person could understand. It allowed the person to grasp the gist. It gave them a sense of control.

Dr. O'Connor offers several cautions for considering these tools. For one, she notes that the shelf life of medical information is growing ever shorter, and that a decision tool based on today's science may be out-of-date tomorrow, no matter how easy it is to use. And she notes that it's important for people to use the right tool at the right time: "It's no use using a decision aid for a stage III disease when you're at stage IV." And she notes that the process of developing decision tools for patients is sporadic and incomplete; for most of us facing medical decisions, having the perfect tool available will be the exception rather than the rule.

But even when the perfect tool isn't available, Dr. O'Connor's work demonstrates that a little mindfulness can go a long way. When somebody is faced with a medical decision, one where there is bound to be uncertainty and doubt and probably will be conflicting recommendations and contradictory science, it's important for us to see a way through the fog, to keep our goals in sight, even if the path is obscured. And when that goal becomes impossible, it's essential that we readjust and set new goals. Health is a series of compromises; we may never be as strong or healthy as we'd like. But knowing how we can optimize our health from where we stand is essential to making the best of what we have.

WHEN CROHN'S DISEASE FORCED Kolya Kirienko to put aside his dreams of going to the Air Force Academy, he was crushed. But within a year, he had a new goal: finish college and go to medical school so he can become a doctor himself. "I'm going to be a gastroenterologist, so I can help people navigate all the stuff that I had to," he says. His condition will sidetrack him along the way, sometimes for months at a time, but he's adamant about getting there. It'll take about 10 years, he figures.

In the meantime, Kolya is putting his computer savvy to work and developing an information-management tool for people with Crohn's to help them manage the reams of data the disease creates (and the intensive decision making it demands). He calls it CrohnologyMD. "It'll grab your lab values and let you know what the results are and what sort of implications they have—do you need a vitamin shot, [need to] adjust your medications, and so on. And it'll let Crohn's patients track their own treatment. You'll be able not only to see how you're doing, but you'll see how your doctor is doing in managing your condition."

In other words, he says with a smile, "It'll let people evaluate their caregivers."

When Patients Become Practitioners

Facing Down Chronic Disease with the Power of Collaboration

I.

TODD SMALL WAS STUCK in quicksand again.

It happened, as it always did, on the floor of the Seattle machine shop where he worked. His shift complete, Todd was making the 150-yard walk from his workbench to his car when he realized that his left leg was sinking deep in the stuff. Though this had happened before—it happened nearly every day now—he stopped and glanced down at his feet. His sneakers looked normal, still firmly planted on the shop's concrete floor. But he was stuck, just the same. His brain was sending an electrical pulse saying "walk," but as the signal streaked from his cerebellum down his spinal cord, it snagged on an inflamed spot where the cord's myelin layer had broken down. The message wasn't getting to his hip flexors, or his hamstrings, or his left foot. That connection had been severed by his multiple sclerosis. And once again, Todd was left with the feeling that, as he described it, "I'm up to my waist in quicksand."

For the 400,000 Americans with multiple sclerosis (MS), Todd Small's description will likely ring true. Muscle weakness is a hallmark of the disease, and foot drop—the term for Todd's quicksand feeling—is a frequent complaint. The condition is usually treated, as it was in Todd's case, with Lioresal (baclofen), a muscle relaxant that works directly on the spinal cord by changing the impulses sent to the muscles. Every day for 14 years, he'd taken a single 10-milligram pill. "My neurologist always told me if you take too much, it will weaken your muscles. So I never wanted to go over 10 milligrams." It never seemed to have much effect, but he carried on as best he could.

Todd would've continued just so, had he not logged on to a Web site called PatientsLikeMe. At first, he expected the sort of online community he'd tried and abandoned several times before—one abundant in sympathy and stories, but little practical information. But here he found something altogether different: data.

After choosing a user name and filling out a profile, Todd was asked to list his symptoms and treatments. He entered the 200 milligrams of Provigil (modafinil) he takes daily to fight fatigue. The Tysabri (natalizumab) injection he takes to slow the progress of his disease. And then he clicked on baclofen, and the Web site told him that nearly 200 patients registered at PatientsLikeMe were taking the drug. He clicked again, and up popped a bold bar graph, placing those 200 across a spectrum of dosages. And there it was. Contrary to what his neurologist had told him years ago, 10 milligrams wasn't the maximum dose. In fact, it was at the low end of the scale. "They're taking 30, 60, sometimes 80 milligrams—and they're just fine," Todd recalls. "So it hits me: I'm not taking nearly enough of this drug."

A few days later, Todd asked his neurologist to up his dosage. Now he takes 40 milligrams of baclofen a day. The new dosage didn't cure his foot drop—he uses a cane now—but he found that after 14 years, he could walk to his car without falling into quicksand. "Oh man, I really dreaded that walk," Todd says. "All shift, it'd be in the back of my mind. Am I going to have trouble? Is it going to get me? Now, I almost got it figured it out. I don't struggle like I used to."

There are nearly 50,000 Todd Smalls at PatientsLikeMe, congregating around a dozen or so diseases from MS to fibromyalgia to depression, all contributing their experiences and tweaking their treatments. At first glance the Web site looks like just another kind of Internet community, a MySpace for the afflicted. Members have user names, post pictures of themselves, and post updates and encouragements. As such, it's akin to the chat rooms and online communities that have inhabited the Internet for more than a decade.

But the members of PatientsLikeMe don't just share their experiences anecdotally; they quantify them, granulate them, digitize them, breaking down their symptoms and treatments into hard data. They note what hurts, where, and for how long. They list their drugs and dosages and score how well they alleviate their symptoms. All this gets compiled over time, aggregated and crunched into tidy bar graphs and progress curves by the software behind the Web site. And it's all open for comparison and analysis.

It operates on the same principles of data and openness that have proven so successful for behavior change at Weight Watchers and Nike+. But instead of applying personal metrics and collaboration toward preventing disease, PatientsLikeMe is putting them at the other end of the health span—where we move from predicting or detecting illness to actually managing it, day after day. And in so doing, by telling all and showing all, the members of PatientsLikeMe are creating an unprecedented database that suggests nothing less than the future of health care.

PATIENTSLIKEME STARTED with a single case of amyotrophic lateral sclerosis, or ALS. In 1998, Stephen Heywood, a 29-year-old carpenter, was diagnosed with the disease, a neurodegenerative disorder commonly known as Lou Gehrig's disease, and Jamie Heywood, his older brother, quit his job to find a cure. An MIT-trained mechanical engineer with a knack for neuroscience, Jamie founded the ALS Therapy Development Institute in Cambridge, Massachusetts, and began a radical quest to save Stephen's life. They tried experimental drug therapies, they tried stem cell transplants, and they tried neural implants, each effort building on the previous one. With each therapy and intervention, Jamie took meticulous notes, chronicling everything on his computer. After 6 years, Stephen was among the most documented ALS patients in the world.

The sheer volume of Stephen's data gave Jamie an idea—a notion hatched while he was browsing Match.com, the online dating site. The aspiring sweethearts there had posted troves of information about themselves. They listed their likes and dislikes, their dating histories, their heights and weights, and any number of other details, all to find a perfect match. Jamie realized that a similar tool might be useful for patients like his brother, not for dating, but to find other people with ALS. If patients shared their information, Jamie figured, and they could find someone with a similar symptomatology and disease history, then they might better plot their own courses of treatment and care. And it didn't just have to be for ALS—it could work for any disease.

Jamie tapped his brother Ben, who had also attended MIT and earned his master's in business administration at UCLA, and they recruited Jeff Cole, a college classmate of Ben's who'd spent several years building dot-coms. They started with Stephen's own case history, breaking it down into drug dosages, symptom severities, and so on. In March of 2006, PatientsLikeMe went online as a community for people with ALS like Stephen. Within a few months, the company added communities for MS and Parkinson's disease. In 2008 the company placed its biggest bet on the model of collective experience, opening a mental health community for the millions of Americans with mood disorders.

The PatientsLikeMe Web site aggregates patient information on two levels: First there's a quantitative breakdown of symptoms and dosages, data that the software instantly turns into charts and graphs. Second are the more qualitative forums, where members share advice and provide more nuanced feedback on a certain drug or treatment issue. The site is designed so that relevant data bolster the conversations in the forums, and vice versa. "Our job is to allow a conversation with the computer that will match a conversation between two patients," Jamie explains. "Then we capture that dialogue and turn it into useful, clean data."

Stephen died on the day after Thanksgiving in 2006, just a few months after the Web site debuted. But his profile, under the user name ALSKing101, still contributes to that online dialogue as a valuable body of data. Just consider this example: Like many people with advanced ALS, in his last 3 years Stephen was living in a wheelchair, completely paralyzed and breathing through a mechanical ventilator. One afternoon, his breathing tube snagged and disconnected, and he suffocated while he was sleeping. Such a death isn't unusual for ALS patients. Many PatientsLikeMe members—dozens are on ventilators—have expressed fears about dying that way. Their main concern is that suffocation is a painful, unpleasant way to go.

As it turns out, the PatientsLikeMe community can allay even that fear. At least two other members of the site have, in fact, had their breathing tubes accidentally disconnected and suffocated until they passed out, only to be found and resuscitated just in time. They have, in other words, almost died in just the way Stephen did, in the way so many have feared, but they lived to tell about it. One of these PatientsLikeMe members described it: "Long story short, my vent hose came off in '97 and I was certain I was going to die. I stared at the clock for exactly ten minutes until I got tunnel vision then passed out. Nothing painful, stressful or anxious about it. It was like I just got sleepy and went to sleep. Suffocation was nothing like what I expected. LoL." Obviously, he lived to tell the story. Laugh out loud, indeed.

ADD UP THE 80 MILLION AMERICANS living with heart disease, the 23 million cases of diabetes, the 46 million with arthritis, and so on down the list, and you soon capture most of the country's 300 million citizens. In fact, if you don't have a chronic disease now, odds are you will: 70 percent of Americans will ultimately die of a chronic disease.

The result: Disease management has become a national reality, a common experience that demands uncommon vigilance. This makes a tool like PatientsLikeMe, one that allows patients to manage their diseases with a sophistication and precision that would've been unimaginable just a decade ago, especially powerful. The 50,000 members of PatientsLikeMe, in other words, are beta testers, the vanguard of how we all will care for and treat our diseases. They're not typical patients, waiting for advice from a doctor. They are, rather, copractitioners in treating their conditions and guiding their care, with potentially profound implications. "People who use it will live longer. People who don't, won't," suggests Jamie Heywood. "That's evolution."

As diseases go, ALS and MS are relatively rare afflictions. Mental illness, on the other hand, afflicts a vast swath of the country. Nearly 60 million Americans have a diagnosable mental disorder, according to the National Institute of Mental Health, a population that includes everything from depression to bipolar disorder to anxiety. For Patients-LikeMe, that population represents a huge market, not to mention a potentially lucrative bounty of data related to antidepressants and other mood disorder drugs. The fact that, as discussed in Chapter 8, most drugs for these disorders won't work for any given patient is, if anything, a bonus for the company.

Jamie's brother Ben Heywood, for instance, gets incensed that antidepressants are, at best, 50 percent effective. "Those odds just aren't good enough," he says. "So you try Wellbutrin and after 6 weeks it doesn't work. Then Prozac. Doesn't work. Now what? Where do you go next?" By plugging in to a community of patients sharing their depression histories and treatments, Ben argues, one could readily find a patient with symptoms and a treatment history close to one's own, compare drug regimens, and go straight to the drug that worked. The odds are better, he says, that the same drug will work for you than with the luck-of-the-draw approach most often used for depression.

This, for many patients, is the promise of a community like Patients-LikeMe: better-targeted treatments at an accelerated rate. And it is similarly the promise of the site as a business. The company, which is funded by private equity, eschews advertising; the business model instead seeks to exploit the value of the databank itself. The pharmaceutical industry should be as eager to improve the targeting and efficacy of their treatments as PatientsLikeMe is. After all, sometimes side effects can turn into blockbusters, most famously when Pfizer scientists learned that their angina treatment was causing erections in men, giving rise to Viagra. What's more, PatientsLikeMe could readily discern which drugs work better for which subpopulations of patients. Such information could be used for what's called drug rescue, when drug companies find new uses for treatments that had been abandoned due to side effects across larger populations. In other words, PatientsLikeMe could pave the way for truly effective pharmacogenomics, helping to create the kind of personalized medicine the drug industry has long promised.

PATIENTSLIKEME IS LOCATED about a mile from the Heywoods' MIT alma mater, in a former twine factory in Cambridge. With about 30 employees, the company is very much a lean operation. Jeff Cole, 38, manages the site's design and software team; Ben, 38, handles overall operations and management; and Jamie, 42, is the frenzied visionary, ever eager to sketch out how powerful a database of 40,000 patient profiles can be.

When I visited the office one fall afternoon, Jamie turned to a nearby whiteboard and traced out an *x-y* axis, slashing a descending line from the upper left to the lower right. "We have the ability to run a probability engine," he said. "We can mathematically model each patient. We can tell them what's going to happen in their life. We can tell you when you'll need a wheelchair," and he made a mark along the line. "And we can even tell you the day you'll die, with remarkable certainty."

Part of Jamie's spiel is bravado. The company doesn't, in fact, predict specific patients' prognoses (though it has filed for a patent covering such prediction tools and has a working prototype). But Jamie's thirst for precision points up the difference between PatientsLikeMe and other companies offering health information and patient communities on the Internet. No other Web site provides information on such a granular scale, nor does any community site aggregate and share members' experiences so rigorously. Indeed, PatientsLikeMe will disappoint someone looking for basic information about a disease; it is not a general resource. But for the patient coping with the cascade of day-to-day decisions that come with managing a disease, it's an unparalleled tool.

II.

THE FIRST THING MANY PEOPLE think of when they hear about a site like PatientsLikeMe—or, for that matter, about any of the data-gathering and tracking tools discussed in this book—is privacy. How can people put such highly personal information—details about their depression, their sex drives, their constipation—out there so openly? Aren't they worried that somebody could use it against them? For that matter, aren't they just *embarrassed*?

The shame of disease, the stigma around it, has been a side effect since leprosy and mental illness caused fear in ancient times. As Susan Sontag wrote back in 1978 in *Illness as Metaphor:* "Any disease that is treated as a mystery and acutely enough feared will be felt to be morally, if not literally contagious." The antidote to such stigma, Sontag suggested, is "to de-mythicize" disease, to reject the fear and the veils of metaphor and stare it down as something real. But that's not so easy. The myths surrounding disease are hard to dispel, our impulse to hide in metaphor difficult to avoid. We still talk of "wars" on cancer and "plagues" of lawyers. "Leper" endures as a metaphor for stigma, long after leprosy itself was eliminated from most of the world. The stigma surrounding disease is hard to shake.

In fact, stigma plays a significant role in the constant concerns over medical privacy. Groups like the World Privacy Forum and Patient Privacy Rights make great hay over the risks of our medical information falling into the wrong hands, pointing especially to fears over electronic medical records. But aside from the financial information contained in those files—which could indeed be misused—by and large the greatest risk these groups can cite comes down to unauthorized disclosures of a condition or a treatment and the potential for embarrassment. In other words, stigma.

It's true that electronic records are a huge challenge to privacy. For decades, our personal health information had been protected largely by sheer chaos, says Mark Rothstein, JD, a bioethics and health policy professor at the University of Louisville, who's an expert in the perils and promise of electronic records. But now, with major health maintenance organizations and hospitals finally moving to adopt electronic health records and companies like Microsoft and Google encouraging the use of personal health records, fallow storerooms of paper records are being converted into neat and portable digital form. And the pace of change makes observers like Rothstein nervous. "Technology is racing ahead of society," he warns. "If this is sensitive information—sexual history, mental illness, substance abuse—even if nothing bad happens, people are subject to stigma and embarrassment."

The federal government has tried to protect patient privacy, most notably with the Health Insurance Portability and Accountability Act, or HIPAA. First enacted in 1996 to help streamline the adoption of electronic records, HIPAA was modified in 2002 to address growing concerns over how those records might be misused or distributed to unauthorized persons. The law stipulates 18 categories of personally identifiable information that must be stripped from records before they may be transferred for commercial or research purposes.

Not surprisingly, HIPAA satisfies no one: not the privacy advocates who argue against most any form of electronic record or the medical researchers who now face onerous restrictions on their work. PatientsLikeMe, though, upends this dialectic; in technology terms, it routes around the problem. Since the company is an opt-in service and not a health care provider, HIPAA doesn't apply (a good thing, really, since the site identifies members' cities and their ages, which are 2 of the 18 categories of personal information HIPAA prohibits revealing).

But HIPAA is extraneous not just legally but also philosophically. Many PatientsLikeMe members volunteer even *more* information from those 18 prohibited categories. They post not only their photos but also photos of their kids and spouses. They add mini-autobiographies and describe their conditions in precise details, including potentially embarrassing particulars on such things as sexual function, bladder control, and constipation. And though they all have user names, most know each other by their first names on the site's forums.

PatientsLikeMe's privacy policy clearly states that this sharing carries risks. It acknowledges that since anybody can register at the Web site, anybody can look at member profiles. And it makes clear that there's no guarantee that another registered member is, in truth, who she says she is. And it nods to the fact that, yes, this is a business, not a public service, and therefore some personally identifiable information may be sold to "approved vendors." But this is boilerplate stuff. The truly subversive notice is the company's Openness Philosophy, a manifesto posted prominently on the site.

"Currently, most healthcare data is inaccessible due to privacy regulations or proprietary tactics," it declares. "As a result, research is slowed, and the development of breakthrough treatments takes decades. . . . When you and thousands like you share your data, you open up the healthcare system. . . . We believe that the Internet can democratize patient data and accelerate research like never before."

This is revolutionary stuff, and it's a new way of thinking about our health information. Instead of being protective of it, instead of looking for ways to lock it up, PatientsLikeMe encourages us to exploit it, to see what we can do with it, how much insight we can gain from it. Instead of being embarrassed that we have a disease or condition, PatientsLikeMe encourages us to accept it—and then to make the most of it.

In 1990, Alan Westin, PhD, an economist at Columbia University, broke Americans into three classes based on their attitudes toward privacy. At one end of the spectrum were what he called the Privacy Fundamentalists, the 25 percent of Americans who felt that their privacy was sacred and that no one, not the government or corporations or their families, should have access to their personal information without explicit permission. At the other end of the spectrum were the Privacy Unconcerned—about 18 percent of Americans—who paid no mind to privacy issues and didn't figure they had anything to hide in any event. In the middle were the vast majority, the 57 percent whom Dr. Westin called the Privacy Pragmatists, those who felt that privacy was a tradeoff. They were willing to give up some information—their birth dates, their ZIP codes, their medical histories—for particular benefits.

In the 20 years since Dr. Westin first offered his taxonomy, the exact percentages have shifted around a bit, but the segments have pretty much held true. But when I spoke to him, Dr. Westin did note that something had changed. It wasn't so much people's feelings about privacy, but rather their relationships to their own information. Where previously only companies or some government agency might find something useful in their personal information, these days individuals can actively exploit their own personal information for specific strategic benefits. The vehicle for that change is the Internet and Web sites like Facebook, Match.com, and PatientsLikeMe. "It's a different world," Dr. Westin says. "People get so much value that they're willing to risk more. They see very direct benefits."

At places like PatientsLikeMe, our information has a currency that's far more liquid than ever before. Converted into data and aggregated with information from others like us, our private information can be invested for both immediate gains and long-term returns. This is the power of sharing. This is the power of openness.

III.

WHEN PEOPLE ARE DIAGNOSED with chronic diseases, they tend to react in one of a few ways. For some there's relief, because they're finally getting a diagnosis, an explanation for what's wrong with them. Others withdraw, surrendering to the idea that their lives are over or ending. Some people, though, engage with their diagnoses. They become self-made experts in their diseases, studying the physiology, the promising treatments, the work of the leading researchers and specialists. They opt for action instead of resignation—and these are the kind of people who find PatientsLikeMe to be such a valuable tool.

There is a historical precedent for people dramatically engaging with their diseases this way. It happened in the 19th century with tuberculosis (TB).

In the 1800s, TB was the great scourge of society. In the United States, as in most of Europe, it was the leading cause of death, accounting for one in five fatalities. Tuberculosis knew no social or racial boundaries, afflicting the old and young and rich and poor alike. But unlike other fatal infectious diseases, TB doesn't bring a quick death. It prefers to linger, leaving its human hosts alive for years and often decades before dispensing with them. (It was, in this sense, the first chronic disease.)

At the beginning of the 19th century, to have tuberculosis (or consumption, as it was then called, an apt description of the way it consumed people from within) was to be an invalid for years on end. It was an exhausting disease, and most people became passive as they counted the days (and often years) till the disease won out. Indeed, this passivity became something of a fashion, with poets and painters imbuing the disease with a romantic shade. Wasting away was simply how consumption was done.

But in the United States around midcentury, that mind-set began to change. With the pioneer spirit aflame in the country, people with TB began to head west, joining the mass migration westward. But instead of land or fortune, they went in search of drier air, warmer weather, and some amount of better health. These were the "health seekers," an army of tuberculars who saw action as their best hope for a cure. In many ways, the health seekers didn't just join the movement westward, they drove it. One-quarter of California immigrants circa 1900 were there because of their health; in Colorado, health seekers constituted one-third of the immigrants. Towns like El Paso, Texas, Colorado Springs, Colorado, and Pasadena, California, were founded and populated by consumptives who thought a new environment would give them new health.

In picking up and moving west the health seekers weren't just pioneers in the cowboys-and-Indians sense. They were pioneers in that they chose to uproot their lives in the hope of achieving better health elsewhere. For decades the health seekers headed west, as many as 7,000 a year, a migration that lasted for nearly 50 years. The movement had such a visible effect on the country that Mark Twain felt it suitable for parody in *Roughing It*, his 1871 narrative of Western escapades. "I know a man who went there to die but he made a failure of it," he says of one consumptive traveler. "He was a skeleton when he came and could barely stand. . . . Three months later he was sleeping out of doors regularly, eating all he could hold, three times a day, and chasing game over mountains three thousand feet high for recreation. And he was a skeleton no longer, but weighed part of a ton. This is no fancy sketch, but the truth."

Truth Twain's tale may not be, but certainly the spirit was true enough. The idea of moving west to find better health became so popular that it wasn't long before land speculators and entrepreneurial physicians and all sorts of others began to work their angles on the health seekers. The movement was truncated only by the discovery of the tuberculosis bacterium in 1882. With Robert Koch's discovery that tuberculosis was a contagion passable from person to person, health seekers suddenly became a lot less welcome out west. Soon, the new domain for treatment was the sanatorium, a quarantined, highly medicalized environment that helped cut down on the spread of disease, but didn't really help those who already had TB; it wasn't until the discovery of antibiotics in the 1940s that TB could be cured.

In retrospect, the health seekers' trek may have been misguided. They were acting on the best available advice, but they were ultimately wrong. But without an alternative, their embrace of action instead of invalidism illustrates how deep our need for control in the face of disease can run. Today, almost 150 years after the health seekers began crossing the continent in search of better health, they serve as a useful example of the power of patient action in the face of chronic disease. After all, even if they didn't find their cures, people with tuberculosis did help forge a nation. Who knows what the millions of people with chronic diseases, computers, and real science might accomplish today.

THESE DAYS, people with chronic diseases don't have to move across the country in search of better air. But they are faced with constantly tending to and managing their diseases. Today, disease management, as it's coldly called, has emerged into a full-blown industry all its own, paralleling the growth of chronic disease. Billions of dollars are spent in the United States alone on helping people tend to chronic conditions; much of this involves simply coping with the diseases. But as the health seekers demonstrated nearly 150 years ago, chronic disease can be met with more than coping. When individuals take charge of their own health, they can be rewarded for changing their habits and adopting activist mind-sets rather than resigning themselves to invalidism.

Of course, one difference (among many) between the 19th-century West and today is that managing one's disease is now a far more complicated proposition. Indeed, one chronic condition often tumbles into another in a series of increasingly dangerous diseases known as comorbid conditions. People with physical disabilities are prone to obesity. People with obesity are prone to diabetes. People with diabetes are prone to develop heart disease. People with heart disease are prone to have strokes. And so on, until death.

Comorbidity is a wonderful term, in its way, sounding at once clinically efficient and slightly spooky. But really, it is a slow and draining process (depression is among the most frequent comorbid conditions accompanying chronic disease, which isn't really surprising, since it is understandably depressing to have a chronic disease). The ultimate result is a treatment regimen that often involves a chaos of pills and shots and doctors' appointments. Managing chronic disease effectively is a job that makes homesteading on the Colorado frontier sound almost easy.

Like the complicated matrix of DNA and disease discussed in Chapters 2 and 3, chronic diseases create their own matrices of conditions and treatments. Every individual comes with his or her own unique hodgepodge of conditions that, in turn, create unique circumstances, needs, and treatments. It's the irony of chronic disease these days: Though nearly everybody's doing it (remember, 70 percent of Americans will die of a chronic disease), there is no template for dealing with it. "It's so obvious that the model for dealing with chronic disease is inadequate," says Stephen Downs of the Robert Wood Johnson Foundation (RWJF), an innovative group that's trying to push our health care system into the 21st century. "In real life you deal with complicated, messy patients. People don't just have diabetes. They have other things going on. Everybody's health is unique. People are complex."

Downs isn't just complaining. For the past 5 years, his group has been working on a new kind of personal health record, one that helps channel the chaos of our medical information into a coherent and *useful* database. With this database, called Project HealthDesign, the

The Cascade of Comorbidity

One chronic disease often leads to another. Obesity, for instance, can lead to dozens of more serious conditions, from depression to heart disease.

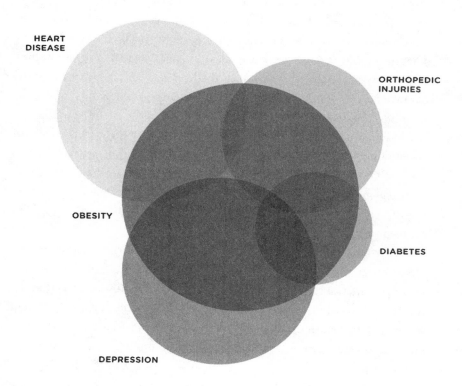

HEART DISEASE

ORTHOPEDIC INJURIES

OBESITY

DIABETES

DEPRESSION

RWJF has set upon the goal of remaking our health information system so the medical record reflects a patient's needs and goals rather than a hospital's or insurance company's.

There has, of course, been plenty of talk over the years about electronic health records. Most systems simply seek to turn our paper medical records from our doctors' offices and hospital visits into electronic form, the type of reform that bioethicist Mark Rothstein warns us may present privacy problems. The medical establishment has been slow to adopt these systems, arguing that they're expensive and time-consuming (both true, though insufficient, arguments). But Downs and his team see electronic records as much more than just the records from our doctors' offices and lists of our prescriptions. They could, he says, capture the continuum of our health, from the way we sleep to the things we eat. "The episodic approach doesn't work," he says, referring to the visit-by-visit accumulation of information. "Seeing just the data from the doctor's office doesn't seem likely to lead to changes in health. It's not the record; it's what you do with it. So we thought, what if we could create something that gets people really engaged with their health, something that captures the data that's *not* in medical records. A lot of times the data we need to know are things like our diet, our sleep, our mood. This stuff has real power for health."

Downs calls these other details ODLs, short for observations of daily living. The RWJF is now funding half a dozen projects that seek to capture ODLs related to chronic diseases—conditions like Crohn's and diabetes and arthritis—and turn them into useful information. By tracking ODLs, a patient might be able to better manage his or her health problems.

Downs's concept of ODLs should sound familiar. It's the same sort of stuff that Nike is doing with Nike+, the same idea behind Microsoft's HealthVault, and so on. It's living by numbers. The difference is that the RWJF wants to get people tracking their information during a different stage of their health cycle—not when we're trying to ward off disease, but when we're trying to manage it and, hopefully, reduce its impact on our lives.

As with any good idea, other companies are catching on to the power of ODLs. A small biotech company called Proteus Biomedical, for instance, has created a nifty system for capturing and using ODLs for people with chronic diseases. The Proteus system starts with a "smart bandage," a self-tracking sensor that sticks on a person's skin like a nicotine patch. From there it can monitor vital signs like body temperature, respiration, and heart rate. Inside the patch is a little chip that sends the vitals data, via Bluetooth, to a cell phone, and from there it goes to the Internet, where it's stored in the individual's file. The information can then be charted and monitored. It's as effective as being hooked up to a bank of machines in a hospital bed—except the patient doesn't have to be confined to his or her bedroom or even home. What's more, the data can be accessed by anybody the patient gives permission to and viewed on anything from an iPhone to a laptop (it should be like catnip to the Quantified Self crowd discussed in Chapter 1).

So it's mobile, passive, and constant self-tracking. So far, so good. But the real genius of the Proteus system is its ability to monitor whether the patient is taking his or her prescribed medications. In other words, it measures compliance. This second function requires another little sensor—this one no bigger than a grain of salt—that can be embedded in a pill or capsule. When a patient swallows the pill, the sensor detects that it has been ingested and, via the smart patch, sends the data to the Internet and then on to the patient's file. It effectively creates a dosage monitoring system, allowing patients to track whether they're taking all their pills at the right times. And since it's all on the Web, other people—doctors, nurses, family members—can get permission to monitor patients' compliance as well. This feature is a godsend for those who want to be sure their loved ones are accurately taking a complicated lineup of pills at certain times every day.

This whole smart-pill idea may sound like *Fantastic Voyage*, the 1966 Raquel Welch sci-fi movie. But it's actually a completely plausible use of some very affordable technologies. Proteus says that pills including the tiny chips can be manufactured for just pennies apiece. The Food and Drug Administration hasn't yet approved the system, but clinical trials are under way in the United Kingdom.

Whether it's Proteus, the RWJF, PatientsLikeMe, or another system, what's clearly emerging here is a new approach to disease management. People facing years of living with chronic diseases don't have to resign themselves to a steady decline into chaos. They don't have to feel they've failed, that they've missed their chances to help their health. With a little smart tracking and collaboration, they can monitor their care, choose their treatments, and make sense of what they're supposed to be doing. They can gain some measure of control over their diseases, and their health.

After all, let's be honest: Most people don't actually start minding their health until they've been diagnosed with something like diabetes or heart disease or some other chronic disease—until, in other words, what we usually think of as being too late. Except it isn't too late. The tools that are emerging mean that even people with chronic diseases can be mindful of their health in ways that improve their prospects. A health system that captures this data stream and combines it with other data might not only make it easier to engage patients in their care, it might turn them from passive observers into health seekers.

IV.

THOUGH TODD SMALL THOUGHT his new dosage of Lioresal helped, it didn't change the trajectory of his disease. He knew that his walking wasn't getting better. It started getting worse. He could feel his mobility slipping away. He hated not being able to dance with his wife. He hated not being able to go to his son's baseball games and walk onto the field. And this time, more Lioresal or another drug wasn't going to help. "The clock is ticking," he told me. "I'm stuck using this cane, and I'm not seeing a lot of improvement in my gait. What I worry about is, the longer I don't walk correctly, the more I'll forget how to walk."

Then he heard about an experimental stem cell treatment for MS. It sounded promising—something about using your own stem cells to rebuild your myelin. But Small, who admits he's no whiz at science, couldn't make out what the research was saying. So he turned to the PatientsLikeMe community. "If somebody could decode this into simple layman's terms, it would be much appreciated," he posted in an online forum.

Small's post kicked off a flurry of collaborative research, with people contributing links to research projects going on in Israel, Finland, and the United Kingdom. Others with a more scientific bent started reading the stuff and synthesizing the bottom line. Skeptics weighed in with questions, and their concerns were met with the firsthand feedback of actual patients who'd undergone the procedure.

Within a few days, Small had his answer. The consensus seemed to point toward research being done by Shimon Slavin, MD, an Israeli physician and the scientific and medical director at the International Center for Cell Therapy and Cancer in Tel Aviv. Dr. Slavin is working on a therapy that uses a patient's own stem cells to treat MS. The process begins by extracting 400 milliliters—a little more than a can of soda—of bone marrow from the leg. In a lab, the marrow is cleaned to isolate the mesenchymal stem cells, which have regenerative properties. For several weeks, those cells are used to grow more cells, after which the patient returns and about 50 million cells are injected into the spinal column. The cells seem to repair some of the damaged myelin in the central nervous system. About 60 patients had been treated with the procedure, and 55 had reported major improvements in their symptoms, including a former Canadian golf pro who was able to return to the game.

It sounded like just what Small had been searching for—a way to take back some of the ground he'd lost to MS. But it was expensive. Small would have to pay $28,000 for his treatment, plus another several thousand dollars to make the trip. Then, one afternoon his wife came home and asked him what he thought about buying a new Buick SUV.

"Yeah, it's nice," Small replied. "We could get a Buick SUV. Or I could get this stem cell treatment." His wife quickly agreed.

"It was a no-brainer," Small told me later. "I just gotta go for it. If I don't do this, I'll be kicking myself. And in another year, I'll have to quit my job at the shop. I have a family. I have two kids. I owe it to them to at least try this."

In June 2009, he and his family boarded a plane headed for Israel to begin the treatment. Three months later, the procedure was complete. Small was getting his strength back and was optimistic that the transplant had worked. But there was still a long road ahead.

SUCH SELF-GUIDED RESEARCH unnerves the medical establishment. That way, they warn, quickly leads to quack cures and dangerous treatments. That's no doubt true in many arenas. But the power of PatientsLikeMe is that its members take their science seriously. They demand published research, not anecdotes. They're quick to debunk phony cures and quackery. They consider themselves not just beneficiaries of research, but participants in an ongoing research project.

In November 2007, a bit of news ricocheted through the PatientsLikeMe ALS community. Researchers in Italy, word had it, appeared to have found that high doses of lithium seemed to slow or even halve the progression of ALS. The Italian study hadn't actually been published, but within 2 months 34 PatientsLikeMe ALS members—nearly twice the number of ALS patients in the Italian study—had lithium prescriptions from their doctors. Just like that, they'd formed an ad hoc clinical trial of lithium. Two years later, nearly 400 ALS patients have tracked their use of lithium on the Web site, using the data tools to chart their progress (140 of them stopped taking the drug). So far, the evidence has failed to replicate the Italian study's findings—results that company scientists have presented at a major ALS conference. But regardless of how well lithium may work, the experiment demonstrates that the Web site quickly outstripped the official study in terms of the volume and detail of information being gathered and tracked.

For his part, Jamie Heywood makes it clear that PatientsLikeMe isn't encouraging ALS members to start taking lithium or encouraging any members to embark on personal experiments. But he's unmistakably excited by the endeavor. As he sees it, the lithium experiment perfectly illustrates how PatientsLikeMe might complement large-scale and long-term clinical research by conducting smaller observational research "on the fly." Jamie calls this "personalized research." And it has a certain logic, at least for those with serious diseases. For those who already have ALS, traditional science works at far too plodding a pace. "The system is broken for terminally ill patients. It makes us wait 5 to 7 years for results when we don't even have that time," says Hanns Riederer, a music producer in Los Angeles who joined the group of ALS members taking lithium. "Even if it's half true, it's still groundbreaking. I don't want to wait for something else. I don't have time to wait."

The lithium experiment testifies to how Web sites like Patients-LikeMe are turning patients into something more—they're becoming self-experimenting amateur scientists. On a smartly run, well-organized Web site, patients can play a huge role in informing each other; they can decentralize and distribute information that once was available only through a personal physician. This means that people can share not only their stories but also best practices and results. The crowd can create its own research, becoming what Jamie describes as "an insight engine."

And it's not just PatientsLikeMe. Collaborative research is likewise a component of CureTogether, a Web site that lets people with dozens of conditions, from allergies to vulvar vestibulitis, track their treatments and symptoms. Like PatientsLikeMe, CureTogether has an insatiable appetite for tracking patient data, and a faith in collaborative insight. The difference lies in the degree to which CureTogether allows patients to control the site. Where PatientsLikeMe taps experts to meticulously design its disease communities, ensuring that the symptomatology and treatments reflect the best thinking on the disease, CureTogether is a much more generic platform. "We let the users have whatever they want," says Alexandra Carmichael, a former computational biologist who founded the site with her husband, Daniel Reda. "It's driven by the patients, not by scientists." That flexibility means the CureTogether platform scales easily across dozens of diseases, with nearly 300 diseases being tackled in the company's first year. Carmichael calls the insights that result from the 5,000 members at CureTogether "collective wisdom."

Sure, some of the insights about these conditions can be somewhat mundane or even spurious. The fact that 77 percent of people with acid reflux say that Tums makes them better is no revelation. And 43 percent of people with acne say it's due to anemia—really? But others are truly remarkable, such as the insights related to the condition that Carmichael herself suffers from, vulvodynia. Vulvodynia is a condition characterized by persistent pain—burning, itching, soreness—in a woman's pelvis and genitals. It can be intermittent or constant, and it makes many aspects of day-to-day life, including sex, seem almost impossible. Despite the fact that as many as 16 percent of women will suffer from it during their lives, it is a woefully understudied condition.

More than 300 women with vulvodynia have found each other at CureTogether, and they have added enough data to yield all sorts of collective wisdom. The most effective treatment seems to be antidepressants and lidocaine, along with some simple behaviors like pelvic floor exercises and not wearing underwear. Lanacane and antibiotics, on the other hand, seem to actually make things worse. Indeed, enough insight has been gathered that the company put together all the research and published a book on the subject.

For Carmichael, whose struggles with vulvodynia helped inspire her to create CureTogether, the information the site has generated about the condition is especially gratifying, since she herself has struggled for so long to understand what was going on in her body. She first had symptoms in 1996 at age 20 and then spent the next decade going to various doctors, hoping they'd have a clue about the source of her pain. She went through endless tests, including an ultrasound to rule out polycystic ovary syndrome and blood panels to rule out hypothyroidism, adrenal fatigue, and a high testosterone level. Time after time, everything turned up normal. No one had any suggestions. Along the way, she had gotten married and had two children.

Finally, in 2006, a new doctor gave her a firm diagnosis: vulvodynia. "It was a huge validation that it was not all in my head, that there was actually a name for what I had, and other women that had it," Carmichael recalls. "It freed me up to focus on how to treat my body rather than try to figure out what I had. It allowed me to connect with other patients. It motivated me to try to help other people with vulvodynia and other undiagnosed chronic pain conditions."

Carmichael's own experience was characterized by a constant struggle with false leads and bad information—exactly what she hopes CureTogether can help eliminate. "It took me 10 years to find out what I had, and it took 2 years to find the right treatment. I just wanted some ideas, some clue, some information. But there wasn't any that I could find," she says. "That simply wouldn't be the case anymore. It would not take anywhere near that long if somebody finds CureTogether. Now there's 300 women like me, sharing ideas and data. It shortens the Decision Tree considerably."

IN 2001, THE AMERICAN MEDICAL ASSOCIATION (AMA) noticed that Americans were using the Internet for health information—and it told them to stop it. "Trust your physician, not a chat room," the AMA suggested in a list of New Year's resolutions. People who use the Internet to self-diagnose and self-medicate, the AMA warned, "may be putting their lives at risk."

Alexandra Carmichael's Decision Tree

It took Alexandra Carmichael 10 years of doctor's visits, Googling, and wrong diagnoses before she found what was responsible for her severe vaginal pain—a condition called vulvodynia. And then it took her another 2 years of trial and error—through a range of alternative therapies—to find relief from the pain. Eventually, she found that the right dosage of hormone replacement therapy offered her the relief she so desperately needed. Here's what that process looks like.

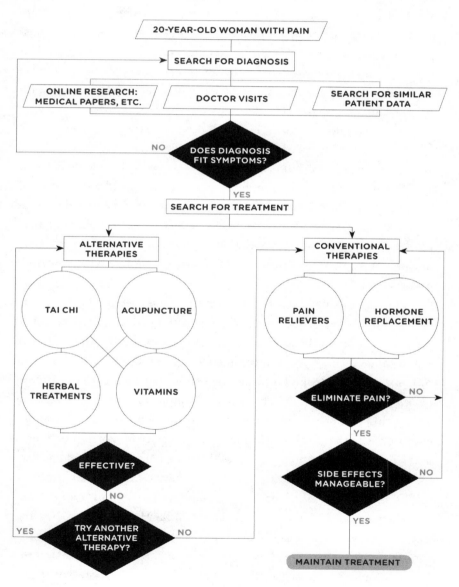

But it's just as absurd to avoid information on the Internet as it is to believe everything on it. PatientsLikeMe could be seen as a direct challenge to physicians' omniscience: The company not only lets members track their disease progression curves, it tacitly encourages them to take action and try to turn those progression curves in a positive direction. While PatientsLikeMe advises patients to consult their doctors before changing their treatments or dosages—they can even print out exhaustive status reports, replete with graphs and charts, to give to their doctors, and personal physicians can register as caregivers on the site—there will inevitably be patients who mistake the Web site's rigor and depth for a substitute for a physician's training and expertise.

Of course, not all collective wisdom is actually smart—especially when it comes to health, and especially on the Internet. Get pulled into an antivaccine vortex online and it's easy to see why. Recommendations and "science" are tossed around like confetti. Groups like the National Vaccine Information Center have set up provocative and compelling Web sites that aim to dissuade parents from vaccinating their children, ignoring the overwhelming evidence that proves vaccines are safe and effective in eliminating horrible diseases. This isn't the wisdom of the crowd; it's mass hysteria.

The aim of this book, though, isn't to praise technology in all its forms and functions. Just as it's foolish of the AMA to cast the entire Internet as a dubious source of information, it would be absurd to say that technology is always a force for good. In fact, I've tried to show that too much technology and information can be detrimental to our overall health. My objective, rather, has been to point toward specific trends and approaches that help us selectively use information to elevate sound science in a way that's relevant, to bring this science closer to individuals and to make it something we can all take advantage of without always having to go through intermediaries and experts.

Of course, not all of these approaches are right for everyone. Constant self-tracking of the sort that PatientsLikeMe requires—updating one's symptoms and dosages and progress—can be tedious, especially for somebody who already has a chronic illness. And not everyone is the "early adopter" type, the kind who's most likely to try a new Web site that asks us to reveal so much about ourselves. But the truth is, you don't have to be an early adopter to understand the virtues of mindfulness.

At their best, Web sites like PatientsLikeMe and CureTogether offer a true middle path—one that has a grounding in science, yes, but also an understanding that we ordinary folk tend to look to each other, rather than textbooks or research papers, for advice on how to lead and improve our lives. The stories we share about our lives, especially stories about our health, can be incredibly influential. Stories matter, and ignoring that fact and insisting on a purely statistical or science-based approach to health care will force many people—maybe most people—to revert toward the traditional doctor-centric mode of medicine. The key is to combine our affinity for stories and narrative with our capacity for rational decision making. It's a combination I've used myself, often, in writing this book. For as much as I have relied on the evidence and published research, most of the chapters in this book begin with stories from people's lives.

In matters of health, the virtue of stories is that they contain information. The opportunity offered by collaboration, the power of collective wisdom, is to organize that information and turn it from dross into better decisions. And better decisions, as I hope I've shown, means better lives.

Coda

When There Is No Doctor:
What Patient-Centric Medicine Really Means

NOW I CAN SAY IT: None of this is new. For years, there's been talk about giving individuals more power over their health care and about using technology to help them make better decisions.

As far back as the 1960s, Warner Slack, MD, a physician and visionary pioneer of personalized medicine, developed a computerized interview tool for incoming patients at the University of Wisconsin. As patients typed in the answers to basic questions about their medical history (of the "Have you ever had an allergic reaction to penicillin?" variety), the computer would monitor their heart rates and their speeds of response, adjusting the questions depending on how they were physically reacting to the interviews. "The largest and least used resource in medicine is the patient," says Dr. Slack, who's now on the faculty at Harvard Medical School. "The idea was to make patients more involved in their care. After all, the patient is the sole subject matter expert on themselves."

If this sounds radical today, it was downright heresy at the time. In a conference on diagnostic medicine in 1970, Dr. Slack presented his vision of computer-enabled "patient power" to a stunned audience of physicians. "The computer can model the physician," Dr. Slack said, suggesting that the patient—not the doctor—should direct his or her own care. "Patients will *not* have to learn clinical medicine, but they will have to know what to expect from the various plans of action offered by the doctor," he told the crowd. (For complex decisions like surgery, Dr. Slack suggested breaking down the process into a "step-by-step evaluation" that sounds very much like a Decision Tree.) And then, provocatively, he added: "Reliance on doctors can be unlearned."

But there's been one persistent obstacle to such scenarios: physicians themselves. Not long before Dr. Slack began programming his computers, a 1961 survey of US surgeons asked whether they routinely shared diagnoses of cancer with their patients. A stunning 90 percent said that no, they wouldn't ordinarily discuss such matters with their patients. This shouldn't come as a great surprise; at the time, Dr. Slack recalls, doctors had an entirely different vocabulary to use in the presence of patients, one that deliberately obscured what may have been wrong. They were trained to say "supratentorial" (referring to a part of the brain) instead of "psychological," and they spoke of "mitotic bodies" instead of cancer. "Doctors used to write prescriptions in Latin to prevent a patient from understanding what they were taking," Dr. Slack says. "The fear was that this information could be dangerous to the patient."

Even 30 years later, in 1991, a survey of physicians in London found that they were unanimous in their concern over giving patients access to their own health records. Such disclosure might "strip away the veneer of medicine," one physician argued, perhaps exposing doctors as charlatans.

Those attitudes sound entirely out of touch today, reflective of a different mind-set and the different values of a different era. And indeed, the trend has reversed among physicians, with nearly all doctors these days in favor of informing patients of their conditions and giving patients access to their records (though these should hardly be controversial propositions). Though some would no doubt still blanch at Dr. Slack's patient-power scenario, most doctors today have been trained to recognize the importance of a patient's wishes under the rubric of "patient autonomy."

But the fact remains that physicians are lagging indicators of change. Doctors, to be sure, have their reasons: They come from a culture of caution and skepticism, in part because conflicting research comes out all the time, and it takes years for consensus to build. Nonetheless, if we really want to empower individuals with authority over their health, history tells us that physicians will not take us there on their own. It is, rather, consumer groups, patients themselves, and sheer economics that are pushing health care toward individuals and away from a doctor-centric model. It's not that physicians don't want the best for their patients; they do. But there's a persistent paternalism in the profession, a fretting over how capable ordinary people are of understanding medical information and acting on their own behalf. A 2007 survey of primary care physicians, funded by the Robert Wood Johnson Foundation, found that most were unprepared for patient-driven medicine, and nearly all were skeptical of the health information patients receive from government or insurance company Web sites (which is somewhat ironic, considering that insurers and their actuarial tables invented the idea of evidence-based medicine). Such opinions reflect the strong conservative tradition in medicine, one that puts faith in the physician above all else. In medicine, paternalism isn't a dirty word; it's the default mode.

But there's conservatism and then there's obstructionism. Some physicians are downright hostile to the notion of their authority being challenged or their decisions second-guessed. Witness the resistance of the American Medical Association (AMA) to putting patients' reviews of doctors online.

In recent years, transparency has come to most every profession, even the most secretive—real estate agents, auto mechanics, even lawyers. All of these have shuddered in the sunlight cast by public review Web sites like Angie's List or Yelp, which solicit opinions from ordinary consumers. Health care is among the last industries to experience this openness, and the idea of public reviews makes the medical establishment exceedingly nervous. Many doctors abhor the idea that people can comment on a doctor's care—often doing so anonymously—and they've often tried to stop these sites from including doctors in their ratings.

But the tide of transparency is becoming harder to stop. In 2006, the Center for the Study of Services, a nonprofit that runs a Web site called Consumers' Checkbook, submitted a Freedom of Information Act request to the US government requesting the release of claims made to

Medicare and Medicaid, including the names of physicians paid for services. The group's idea was to put the information online in a searchable database, one that people could use to look up whether a doctor was performing according to guidelines. After the government turned down the request, citing physicians' privacy, the group filed suit for the release of the information. The AMA joined the case, arguing that the government should by no means release the data. The doctors' right to privacy, the AMA argued, clearly outweighed the public's right to know about their doctors. In 2007, a lower court told the government to hand over the data. But in 2009, an appeals court overturned that ruling in a split decision. The consumer group is considering a further appeal.

Regardless of what comes of the effort, the fight demonstrates that the paternalism Dr. Slack fought against 40 years ago is still alive and well. And it's often self-justifying paternalism, in that it keeps the AMA and physicians in business as the sole arbiters of medical information. The AMA, I should add, does not speak for all physicians; less than one-third of US doctors belong to the AMA (and as many as half of AMA members are medical students and residents who get a discount on membership). But the group is a powerful force in determining how health care is delivered and has a long record of obstructing change, as demonstrated by its role in helping to defeat FDR's health care reforms in the 1940s and its losing the battle against Medicare in the 1960s.

This time, the AMA may once again be on the wrong side of history. Automation has come to experts of all sorts: stockbrokers, travel agents, financial advisors, and on down the list. This is the very definition of disruption—an entrenched power finding itself isolated and antiquated as a small-scale innovation quietly replaces it.

The fact is that physicians are an overworked lot (though they are rarely underpaid). Their tasks range from keeping files to dealing with insurance companies to—oh, yeah—actually providing care for their patients. Maybe they need a break. Maybe they could use some help. From us.

Let me say here that I come from a family of physicians and health care providers. I have great respect for the vocation; I wouldn't be writing this book if I didn't. But today, when information technology offers so much assistance to people facing health care issues, our health is too important to leave to an archaic, insular, and information-poor structure. If there's no longer a need to rely solely on a doctor's advice for treatment and care, why should we be expected to artificially limit our options?

This is not to say that we don't need doctors and surgeons and nurses for their expertise. We absolutely do. We need them to diagnose us and help us parse information, and we especially need them to execute solutions—to write prescriptions, perform operations, and so on. To repeat: Instead of being the sole interface for all medical information and care, physicians should augment and support our decisions. "People ask me if the computer will replace the doctor," says Dr. Slack of Harvard. "And I've always had the same answer: Any doctor who can be replaced by a computer deserves to be. The open exchange of information with a patient is essential to the successful practice of medicine."

It's likewise important to acknowledge that the health care system is poorly designed to encourage doctors to hew to this new role. As I write this, health care reform appears to be on the horizon in the United States. But simply providing health care insurance and rooting out some inefficiencies won't address the deeper division that has emerged between individuals and the idea of preventive medicine on one side and physicians and the realities of their paychecks on the other side. It's not just a communication problem; there's a systems problem here.

The problems start with how physicians get paid. Physicians are largely compensated for performing specific services, matching a treatment or a diagnosis to its respective billing code. Mark McClellan, MD, PhD, a former commissioner of the Food and Drug Administration and a former administrator at the Center for Medicare and Medicaid Services (known as CMS) described the problem precisely. "We've got a health care delivery system that is organized the wrong way: It provides the wrong services with the wrong emphasis," Dr. McClellan said at a 2008 meeting of the Patient-Centric Leadership Forum. "You can trace this back to the fact that reimbursement is wrong. We have payment incentives that encourage more intensity, especially after a health problem has developed, and don't have any real accountability for getting better results for patients' health at the lowest overall cost. We have systems of choice in our health care system that don't really give people a choice."

This "fee for service" model, though, only works when there's something wrong that must be treated. It's far less effective at compensating physicians for preventive care or keeping patients healthy. This alternative approach—known in policy circles as pay for performance—has made some inroads in recent years, most prominently in health management organizations (it's used on an experimental basis in Medicare, which pays for nearly 20 percent of the health care services delivered in the United States). Pay-for-performance isn't perfect; Jerome Groopman, MD, and Pamela Hartzband, MD, recently argued in the *Wall Street Journal* that "quality metrics" used to rate performance turn hospitals into factories where physicians have little discretion to use their judgment.

But the evidence shows that when it's used, pay-for-performance does indeed change the way medicine is practiced. "Pay for performance has been remarkable in its ability to improve performance," says Peter Bach, MD, of Memorial Sloan-Kettering Cancer Center in New York and a former senior advisor at CMS. Dr. Bach notes that when health plans systematically measure preventive care in the forms of rates of screening, smoking termination, and immunization as well as other metrics, the quality of care routinely improves. "Of course you could look at this as a glass-half-empty scenario, that you have to start measuring something to get care to an acceptable level. That's an affront to my profession, particularly when they're measuring something as stupid as whether docs give patients an aspirin after a heart attack. But the fact is, every place we shine the light we get improvement."

The relative success of pay-for-performance would argue for expanding the approach to accommodate more preventive measures, compensating doctors and mandating insurance coverage for genetic scans, additional routine checkups, and so forth. But the AMA has been vociferous in its defense of fee-for-service as the standard payment method. The AMA loves fee-for-service because it keeps payments for specialists—who account for most of its members—high, since every test is charged for separately.

Again, in the United States, health care reform may well address some of these issues. But ultimately, the true advent of patient power won't happen because of the government, or the AMA, or even your personal physician. The movement to put individuals in charge, and to give them the resources to do it, starts with us.

BUT SHOULD WE WANT PEOPLE TO BE IN CHARGE? Do they even want to be in charge? Certainly, ordinary citizens have a mixed track record on acting in their best interest, as Aristotle made clear with *akrasia* so long ago. People are lazy. They're slow. They can be irrational. Giving people more responsibility over their health, some would argue, is a good way to increase rates of obesity and other behavior-related conditions. After all, about half of patients fail to follow their physicians' orders, and about 40 percent incorrectly follow the directions for their prescriptions (which typically means that they miss doses).

And when they do act, people often choose to do the wrong things— witness the flourishing of sham science, pseudocures, and dubious nutraceuticals. There seems no end of scams that some people will fall for.

So if the evidence says that people sometimes make bad decisions that actually harm them, how can this book advocate more autonomy? In part, I take my cue from Donald Berwick, MD, president of the Institute for Healthcare Improvement, who calls himself an "extremist" when it comes to empowering patients. "'Exceptional cases make bad rules,'" he argued in a resounding 2009 manifesto for patient control. "You do not successfully rebut my plea for extreme patient-centeredness by telling me that, on rare occasions, we ought to say, 'No.' I say, 'Your "rare occasions" make for very bad rules for the usual occasions.'" We need to build a system that gives people autonomy and gives them the tools to get the best results, regardless of the fact that some people will come up short. The opportunity is too great to shortchange the many because of the limitations of a few.

But perhaps more importantly, this is a trend that's happening even without patients'-rights advocates and a few renegade physicians. There are pure economic forces driving patient-centric care as well. The insurance industry is pushing us to take more responsibility for our health by way of our pocketbooks. Individuals are now on the hook for a set fee—known as a co-pay—for every doctor's visit and must routinely pay for a set amount of their medical care—known as a deductible—before insurance kicks in. Since 2003, co-pays and deductibles for patients have been increasing by more than 15 percent per year. The rationale, in part, is that if we're paying for our care, we'll think about what we need—and what we don't—more explicitly. If you want people to think about their health, the logic goes, just ask them to open their wallets.

These fees do, in fact, get people to think twice about how they use medical care. Researchers have found that even small co-pays tend to decrease the so-called moral hazard for patients, leading them to demand less care. And that can be a good thing: As Shannon Brownlee demonstrated in *Overtreated* and as Atul Gawande reminded us in a much-discussed 2009 *New Yorker* article, more care doesn't necessarily correspond to better health, and less care can actually correspond to better outcomes. But it's not clear that these fees are actually getting people to think differently about how *they* can manage their own health, rather than a doctor or hospital. In other words, co-pays and deductibles may be a good stick for dissuading people from using expensive late-stage care. But there still needs to be a carrot that makes self-guided preventive behaviors advantageous.

Other trend lines are pushing toward the same result. Every year in the United States, there are fewer primary care doctors and less time is spent on primary care (many European countries show a similar trend). When patients do get a doctor's visit scheduled, there's increasingly less time spent talking face to face. And, from the other direction, people are spending more time online researching medical information. Patient power is the way things are headed, whether we're ready for it or not.

The decision now before all of us—doctors and laypeople, providers and patients, the ill and the vital, the young and the old—is whether we want to be in the vanguard of this change or dragged along with it. As I've tried to show, there are many reasons to be enthusiastic about the opportunity to make more of our health, and the least of them is that it's happening with us or without us.

In the context of top-down, bureaucratic, economic health care reforms, the Decision Tree approach should be considered the bottom-up corollary, a grassroots movement that can get individuals working toward the shared goals of more prevention, earlier detection, and smarter treatments. Ultimately, that is the message of this book. The tools are out there, now, for individuals to start taking action and secure some measure of control over their health care. And control is everything: It can tip the balance away from illness and toward health. The more we insert ourselves into the decision-making process, the more the results will reflect what we consider to be good outcomes.

For those who remain unconvinced, who would scoff at the notion of patient power like the crowd scoffed at Warner Slack 40 years ago, I can only say this: Look to history. Sooner or later, the public, empowered by technology and motivated by self-interest, tends to prevail. It's folly to underestimate the potential of highly motivated individuals to get things right.

Acknowledgments

I first made the decision to write this book as a student at the School of Public Health at the University of California, Berkeley. As a journalist, I was an odd duck in the SPH pond, but Nap Hosang, the wise and indomitable force behind the interdisciplinary program, not only gave me a slot but became a valuable mentor. He recognized where I was headed before I did. I'm grateful for his guidance.

Many of the ideas in this book were first tested in the pages of *Wired* magazine. I'm grateful to all my colleagues there. Jacob Young, Scott Dadich, Mark McClusky, and Mark Robinson, who edited several pieces integrated into this book, have all been essential partners and friends. Bob Cohn, with whom I had the pleasure of working side by side for over a decade, has been an engaged and curious reader and editor. And Chris Anderson, *Wired*'s editor-in-chief, not only allowed me to play hooky from *Wired,* he took to my ideas and helped carve them into shape. I owe him special thanks for his advice, example, and friendship.

An essential partner along the way was my researcher and co-blogger, Brian Mossop, a successful neuroscientist who for some reason decided to slum with a nonscientist. Brian's pithy, clear dispatches helped me better understand and articulate the ideas in this book, and his humor and patience as I worked through an idea were always welcome. Victor Krummenacher, whose skills with InDesign approach his skills on the bass guitar, took considerable time to craft the nearly 30 charts herein. And Steven Leckart, a model 21st-century journalist, pitched in to research and correct many of my facts. Several journalist friends read the manuscript and offered invaluable critiques, including Robin Sloan, Jeff O'Brien, and Jonah Lehrer. The brilliant Jason Bobe at the Personal Genome Project was exceedingly generous with his ideas and resources. Dr. Ray Dantes, my classmate at Berkeley and now a resident at UCSF, took time to read the book and offer astute advice, as did Dr. Eddie Greene at the Mayo Clinic, a lifelong friend to the whole Goetz clan. Dr. Jodi Halpern at Berkeley's School of Public Health was a source of ideas and support.

There would be no book at all if not for the polymathic mind of Chris Calhoun. My friend before he somehow became my agent, Chris is one of the true wits in the book business. His patience, encouragement, and good humor helped me mold a jumble of ideas into this crisp one. One of Chris's best decisions was to send the proposal to my whip-smart editor, Colin Dickerman, who at the time hadn't even seen his desk at Rodale. Colin's enthusiasm for the project, and his careful and cogent reads, made quick work of what could've been a slog. Colin, Karen Rinaldi, and their team at Rodale are the sharpest crew of booksmiths I've ever met. Their confidence in the book was invaluable in steeling my own.

You don't choose your family, but my parents, Dr. Frederick and Mary Rose Goetz, taught me how to make decisions and supported some ungodly foolish ones along the way. My brother, Fred, taught me the power of argument at a young age. My sister Laura, a surgeon and keen intellect, has been a tremendous resource and friend. She is always generous with encouragement and advice, and I'm consistently proud to be her brother. My sister Cecilia was in many ways the inspiration for this book. I never would have thought of studying public health if not for her example. She was right: It is a great way to look at the world, and I'm forever sorry that she's not here to continue in her work and improve my own.

My most essential critic and biggest supporter has been my wife, Whitney Wright, who not only encouraged me in every pursuit but has been an insightful editor. An expert in group dynamics and behavior change in her own right, Whitney has patiently watched me catch up to what she's known all along. I'm ever grateful for whatever combination of choice, fate, and environment brought us together.

Lastly, I want to give my deep thanks to the individuals whose names and stories appear in this book. They've generously shared their circumstances in the belief that their decisions may better guide others'. I hope this book rewards that gesture.

Notes

Introduction

page ix "In the case of MS, . . . " Nancy J. Holland, T. Jock Murray, and Stephen C. Reingold, *Multiple Sclerosis: A Guide for the Newly Diagnosed,* 3rd ed. (New York: Demos Medical Publishing, 2007).

page xi "In 1910, polio and smallpox . . . " The wondrous story of vaccines, too often taken for granted today, is superbly told in Arthur Allen's *Vaccine: The Controversial Story of Medicine's Greatest Lifesaver* (New York: W.W. Norton, 2007).

page xi "In 1910, diabetes was a horrible disease . . . " Frank N. Allan, "Diabetes Before and After Insulin," *Medical History* 16(1972): 266–273.

page xiv "Indeed, more than 70 percent of the $2 trillion . . . " Centers for Disease Control and Prevention, "Chronic Disease Overview: Costs of Chronic Disease," November 20, 2008. www.cdc.gov/nccdphp/overview.htm.

page xviii "Early detection of ovarian cancer, . . . " Vladimir Nossov, Malaika Amneus, Feng Su, Jennifer Lang, Jo Marie Tran Janco, Srinivasa T. Reddy, and Robin Farias-Eisner, "The Early Detection of Ovarian Cancer: From Traditional Methods to Proteomics," *American Journal of Obstetrics and Gynecology* 199(2008): 215–223.

page xxi "In November 2008, *Operations Research,* . . . " Ralph L. Keeney, "Personal Decisions Are the Leading Cause of Death," *Operations Research* 56(2008): 1335–1347. Also see *Smart Choices: A Practical Guide to Making Better Decisions,* written by Keeney, John S. Hammond, and Howard Raiffa (Boston: Harvard Business School Press, 1999).

Chapter 1

page 4 "In the years after World War II, . . . " The history of and work stemming from the Framingham Heart Study are nicely presented by the National Heart, Lung, and Blood Institute and Boston University at www.framinghamheartstudy.org. For a thorough and readable narrative history of the study, see Daniel Levy and Susan Brink's *A Change of Heart: How the Framingham Heart Study Helped Unravel the Mysteries of Cardiovascular Disease* (New York: Knopf, 2005).

page 6 "It's a pleasant spring evening . . . " The Quantified Self meet up is organized by Gary Wolf and Kevin Kelly, two visionary thinkers and writers, and chronicled at www.quantifiedself.com. Gary's eloquent manifesto on the group's mission was published as "Know Thyself" in *Wired,* July 2009.

page 9 "In 1967, just as the Framingham . . . " Geoffrey Rose and M. G. Marmot, "Social Class and Coronary Heart Disease," *British Heart Journal* 45(1981): 13–19. For the full story on the wonderful Whitehall study and its profound implications, see Marmot's *The Status Syndrome: How Social Standing Affects Our Health and Longevity* (New York: Times Books, 2004). For a taste of the primary research, see M. G. Marmot, G. D. Smith, S. Stansfeld, C. Patel, F. North, J. Head, I. White, E. Brunner, and A. Feeney, "Health Inequalities among British Civil Servants: The Whitehall II Study," *Lancet* 337(1991): 1387–1393.

page 13 ". . . the declining numbers of primary care doctors, . . . " Survey conducted by the Association of American Medical Colleges and the American Medical Association.

page 16 "Kaiser's Maui Lani Clinic . . . " A discussion of the Maui clinic project can be found in Gerard Livaudais, Robert Unitan, and Jay Post, "Total Panel Ownership and the Panel Support Tool—'It's All About the Relationship,'" *Permanente Journal* 10(2006): 72–79. Also see a thorough evaluation by the Agency for Healthcare Research and Quality, "Team-Based Ownership Over Defined Patient Panels Supported by Information Technology Enhances Provision of Evidence-Based Care," April 14, 2008. www.innovations.ahrq. gov/content.aspx?id=1699.

page 18 "For women of a certain age, . . . " Jacques E. Rossouw, Garnet L. Anderson, Ross L. Prentice, Andrea Z. LaCroix, Charles Kooperberg, Marcia L. Stefanick, Rebecca D. Jackson, et al., "Risks and Benefits of Estrogen Plus Progestin in Healthy Postmenopausal Women: Principal Results from the Women's Health Initiative Randomized Controlled Trial," *JAMA* 288(2002): 321–333. *JAMA*'s editorial is Suzanne W. Fletcher and Graham A. Colditz, "Failure of Estrogen Plus Progestin Therapy for Prevention," *JAMA* 288(2002): 366–368.

page 21 "Dr. Schwartz and her husband, . . . " Schwartz and Woloshin have written a helpful book to guide consumers: Steven Woloshin, Lisa M. Schwartz, and H. Gilbert Welch, *Know Your Chances: Understanding Health Statistics* (Berkeley: University of California Press, 2008). For examples of their thorough research, see Steven Woloshin, Lisa M. Schwartz, and H. Gilbert Welch, "Patients and Medical Statistics: Interest, Confidence, and Ability," *Journal of General Internal Medicine* 20(2005): 996–1000. Also useful is Lisa M. Schwartz, Steven Woloshin, and H. Gilbert Welch, "Can Patients Interpret Health Information? An Assessment of the Medical Data Interpretation Test," *Medical Decision Making* 25(2005): 290–300.

page 23 "The Drug Facts box . . . " Schwartz and Woloshin's experiment was published as Lisa M. Schwartz, Steven Woloshin, and H. Gilbert Welch, "The Drug Facts Box: Providing Consumers with Simple Tabular Data on Drug Benefit and Harm," *Medical Decision Making* 27(2007): 655–662.

page 24 "In the 1920s, the Western Electric . . . " Rob McCarney, James Warner, Steve Iliffe, Robbert van Haselen, Mark Griffin, and Peter Fisher, "The Hawthorne Effect: A Randomised, Controlled Trial," *BMC Medical Research Methodology* 7(2007): 30.

page 25 "As it turns out, the story . . . " Steven D. Levitt and John A. List, "Was There Really a Hawthorne Effect at the Hawthorne Plant? An Analysis of the Original Illumination Experiments," National Bureau of Economic Research Working Paper No. 15016, May 2009.

pages 25–26 "A 2006 study in a German hospital . . . " Tim Eckmanns, Jan Bessert, Michael Behnke, Petra Gastmeier, and Henning Rüden, "Compliance with Antiseptic Hand Rub Use in Intensive Care Units: The Hawthorne Effect," *Infection Control and Hospital Epidemiology* 27(2006): 931–934.

page 26 "The experiment started at a Kansas City . . . " Philip H. Feil, Jennifer Sherah Grauer, Cynthia C. Gadbury-Amyot, Katherine Kula, and Michael D. McCunniff, "Intentional Use of the Hawthorne Effect to Improve Oral Hygiene Compliance in Orthodontic Patients," *Journal of Dental Education* 66(2002): 1129–1135.

page 27 "This has been demonstrated, . . . " Meghan L. Burtryn, Suzanne Phelan, James O. Hill, and Rena R. Wing, "Consistent Self-Monitoring of Weight: A Key Component of Successful Weight Loss Maintenance," *Obesity* 15(2007): 3091–3096.

page 28 " 'Filling out that sheet . . . ' " Levy, *A Change of Heart*.

Chapter 2

page 32 "In the late 1970s, a prenatal test . . . " For details on Down syndrome rates in the United States, see James F. X. Egan, Peter A. Benn, Carolyn M. Zelop, Alan Bolnick, Elisa Gianferrari, and Adam F. Borgida, "Down Syndrome Births in the United States from 1989 to 2001," *American Journal of Obstetrics and Gynecology* 191(2004): 1044–1048. For information on worldwide rates since prenatal testing began, see Claire Irving, "Twenty-Year Trends in Prevalence and Survival of Down Syndrome," *European Journal of Human Genetics* 16(2008): 1336–1340.

page 33 "Since 2007, the American College . . . " American College of Obstetricians and Gynecologists, "New Recommendations for Down Syndrome: Screening Should Be Offered to All Pregnant Women," news release, January 2, 2007.

page 34 "A recent study in the *Journal of Pediatrics* . . . " Virginie Scotet, Baroukh M. Assael, Ingrid Duguépéoux, Anna Tamanini, Marie-Pierre Audrézet, Claude Férec, and Carlo Castellani, "Time Trends in Birth Incidence of Cystic Fibrosis in Two European Areas: Data from Newborn Screening Programs," *Journal of Pediatrics* 152(2008): 25–32.

page 34 "Increasingly, life brings other genetic tests . . . " For a thorough perspective from bioethicists on genetics, see Allen Buchannan, Dan W. Brock, Norman Daniels, and Daniel Wikler, *From Chance to Choice: Genetics and*

Justice (Cambridge, UK: Cambridge University Press, 2000). Also worth reading is Michael J. Green and Jeffrey R. Botkin, "'Genetic Exceptionalism' in Medicine: Clarifying the Differences between Genetic and Nongenetic Tests," *Annals of Internal Medicine* 138(2003): 571–575.

page 39 "When Gregor Mendel . . . " Google Books has made available the fifth edition of a fine book by Reginald Crundall Punnett called *Mendelism,* published by Macmillan in London in 1922. It reflects a near-contemporary understanding of his work.

page 44 "Panel after panel . . . " See, for instance, the recommendations of the Alzheimer Disease Working Group of the Stanford Program in Genomics, Ethics, and Society, published as L. M. McConnell, B. A. Koenig, H. T. Greely, and T. A. Raffin, "Genetic Testing and Alzheimer Disease: Has the Time Come?" *Nature Medicine* 4(1998): 757–759.

page 44 "This ambiguity inspired the REVEAL . . . " Robert Green's work has resulted in several notable papers, the most recent of which is Robert C. Green, J. Scott Roberts, L. Adrienne Cupples, Norman R. Relkin, Peter J. Whitehouse, Tamsen Brown, Susan LaRusse Eckert, et al., "Disclosure of *APOE* Genotype for Risk of Alzheimer's Disease," *New England Journal of Medicine* 361(2009): 245–254. Also worth reading with regard to the measures *APOE*-positive individuals take in response to learning their risk is Serena Chao, J. Scott Roberts, Theresa Marteau, Rebecca Silliman, L. Adrienne Cupples, and Robert C. Green, "Health Behavior Changes after Genetic Risk Assessment for Alzheimer Disease: The REVEAL Study," *Alzheimer Disease and Associated Disorders* 22(2008): 94–97.

Chapter 3

page 50 "Curry's diagnosis . . . " Curry's story is compiled from several newspaper accounts, among them Howard Beck, "No Information Yet from Tests, or from Curry," *New York Times,* October 7, 2005.

page 52 "These were the first members . . . " Church has chronicled the project himself, starting with the manifesto "Genomes for All" in *Scientific American,* January 2006. Also see Carey Goldberg, "Personal Genome Project Participants Get First Look at Their DNA," *Boston Globe,* October 20, 2008. The PGP's progress can be tracked at www.personalgenomes.org.

page 56 ". . . even de-identified data are subject . . . " Latanya Sweeney, "k-Anonymity: A Model for Protecting Privacy," *International Journal on Uncertainty, Fuzziness and Knowledge-Based Systems* 10(2002): 557–570.

page 62 "Even the sober *New England Journal* . . . " David J. Hunter and Peter Kraft, "Drinking from the Fire Hose—Statistical Issues in Genomewide Association Studies," *New England Journal of Medicine* 357(2007): 436–439.

page 63 "Within 6 months of 23andMe . . . " Alexis Madrigal, "Meeting Reveals California's Hardline Stance on DNA Testing," *Wired Science,* June 18, 2008. www.wired.com/wiredscience/2008/06/regulator-wants.

page 64 " . . . called the services premature . . . " David J. Hunter, Muin J. Khoury, and Jeffrey M. Drazen, "Letting the Genome Out of the Bottle—Will We Get Our Wish?" *New England Journal of Medicine* 358(2008): 105–107. Also see American Medical Association, "Report 7 of the Board of Trustees: Direct-to-Consumer Advertising and Provision of Genetic Testing," 2008. And see Sarah E. Gollust, Sara Chandros Hull, and Benjamin S. Wilfond, "Limitations of Direct-to-Consumer Advertising for Clinical Genetic Testing," *JAMA* 288(2002): 1762–1767.

page 64 "The medical establishment has been woefully . . . " Erin E. Tracy, Kathy Hudson, Gail Javitt, Wylie Burke, and Peter Byers, "Are Doctors Prepared for Direct-to-Consumer Advertising of Genetics Tests?" *Obstetrics and Gynecology* 110(2007): 1389–1391.

page 65 "David Goldstein, PhD, the director . . . " David B. Goldstein, "Common Genetic Variation and Human Traits," *New England Journal of Medicine* 360(2009): 1696–1698.

Chapter 4

page 70 "With a strong link emerging . . . " Norman Jolliffe, Ethel Maslansky, Florence Rudensey, Martha Simon, and Alice Faulkner, "Dietary Control of Serum Cholesterol in Clinical Practice," *Circulation* 24(1961): 1415–1421.

page 70 "Then 38 years old, Nidetch . . . " Nidetch recounts her struggles with weight loss and her eventual Weight Watchers triumph in her 1970 autobiography, *The Story of Weight Watchers* (New York: W/W Twentyfirst).

page 74 "A 2003 study published in *JAMA*, . . . " Stanley Heshka, James W. Anderson, Richard L. Atkinson, Frank L. Greenway, James O. Hill, Stephen D. Phinney, Ronette L. Kolotkin, Karen Miller-Kovach, and F. Xavier Pi-Sunyer, "Weight Loss with Self-Help Compared with a Structured Commercial Program: A Randomized Trial," *JAMA* 289(2003): 1792–1798.

page 74 "A subsequent study, published . . . " Adam Gilden Tsai and Thomas A. Wadden, "Systematic Review: An Evaluation of Commercial Weight Loss Programs in the United States," *Annals of Internal Medicine* 142(2005): 56–66.

page 75 "A 2004 study found that barely 3 percent . . . " Lawrence J. Fine, G. Stephanie Philogene, Robert Gramling, Elliot J. Coups, and Sarbajit Sinha, "Prevalence of Multiple Chronic Disease Risk Factors: 2001 National Health Interview Survey," *American Journal of Preventive Medicine* 27 Suppl.(2004): 18–24. A thorough and surprisingly readable textbook on behavior change is Sally A. Shumaker, Judith K. Ockene, and Kristin A. Riekert, eds., *The Handbook of Health Behavior Change*, 3rd ed. (New York: Springer, 2009).

page 76 "Back in 350 BC, . . . " Aristotle, *The Nicomachean Ethics* (New York: Penguin, 2004).

page 78 "Titled *Promoting Health:* . . . " Brian D. Smedley and S. Leonard Syme, eds., *Promoting Health: Intervention Strategies from Social and Behavioral Research* (Washington, DC: National Academy Press, 2000).

page 79 "Dr. Syme's favorite example . . . " Jeremiah Stamler and James D.

Neaton, "The Multiple Risk Factor Intervention Trial (MRFIT)—Importance Then and Now," *JAMA* 300(2008): 1343–1345.

page 80 "In the late 1990s, the Centers for Disease Control . . . " National Diabetes Information Clearinghouse, "Diabetes Prevention Program," NIH Publication No. 09-5099, October 2008. http://diabetes.niddk.nih.gov/dm/pubs/preventionprogram.

pages 82–83 "The system is basic self-monitoring, . . . " Albert Bandura, "Self-Efficacy: Toward a Unifying Theory of Behavioral Change," *Psychological Review* 84(1977): 191–215. For more on Bandura's remarkable work, see Richard I. Evans, *Albert Bandura, the Man and His Ideas—A Dialogue* (New York: Praeger, 1989).

page 84 "The recently completed ALIVE . . . " Gladys Block, Barbara Sternfeld, Clifford H. Block, Torin J. Block, Jean Norris, Donald Hopkins, Charles P. Quesenberry, Gail Husson, and Heather Anne Clancy, "Development of Alive! (A Lifestyle Intervention Via Email), and Its Effect on Health-Related Quality of Life, Presenteeism, and Other Behavioral Outcomes: Randomized Controlled Trial," *Journal of Medical Internet Research* 10(2008): e43.

page 84 "It is, as one textbook describes . . . " Barbara S. McCann and Victor E. Boubjerg, "Promoting Dietary Change," *The Handbook of Health Behavior Change,* 3rd ed. (New York: Springer, 2009), 222.

page 85 "Dr. Bandura paved the way . . . " Albert Bandura, Dorothea Ross, and Sheila A. Ross, "Transmission of Aggression through Imitation of Aggressive Models," *Journal of Abnormal and Social Psychology* 63(1961): 575–582.

page 86 "But another body of evidence is emerging . . . " The work of Christakis and Fowler is captured in their recent book, *Connected: The Surprising Power of Our Social Networks and How They Shape Our Lives* (New York: Little, Brown, 2009). For specific study data, see Nicholas A. Christakis and James H. Fowler, "The Spread of Obesity in a Large Social Network Over 32 Years," *New England Journal of Medicine* 357(2007): 370–379; and "The Collective Dynamics of Smoking in a Large Social Network," *New England Journal of Medicine* 358(2008): 2249–2258.

page 90 "The Nike+ sensor consists . . . " *Wired*'s Mark McClusky wrote the definitive story on Nike+ in "The Nike Experiment: How the Shoe Giant Unleashed the Power of Personal Metrics," *Wired,* July 2009. My description of the tool draws on his.

Chapter 5

page 98 "Metabolic syndrome is characterized . . . " A good primer on research into the syndrome is Christopher D. Byrne and Sarah Wild, eds., *The Metabolic Syndrome* (Chichester, UK: John Wiley, 2005).

page 101 "Take the case of Franklin . . . " The story of FDR is a favorite among medical historians because it so clearly illustrates how far we've come in terms of using best practices for risk prevention. Roosevelt's story is thoroughly detailed in Howard G. Bruenn, "Clinical Notes on the Illness and Death of President Franklin D. Roosevelt," *Annals of Internal Medicine* 72(1970): 579–591.

page 102 "Hypertension was the obvious test . . . " My discussion of the histories of hypertension and diabetes draws extensively on Jeremy A. Greene's superb scholarship on risk-based diagnosis in *Prescribing by Numbers: Drugs and the Definition of Disease* (Baltimore: Johns Hopkins University Press, 2008).

page 104 "Each such study potentially . . . " Erin D. Michos and Roger S. Blumenthal, "Prevalence of Low Low-Density Lipoprotein Cholesterol with Elevated High Sensitivity C-Reactive Protein in the U.S.: Implications of the JUPITER (Justification for the Use of Statins in Primary Prevention: An Intervention Trial Evaluating Rosuvastatin) Study," *Journal of the American College of Cardiology* 53(2009): 931–935.

page 104 "'What we see in patients . . . '" Managing Cardiometabolic Risk: Will New Approaches Improve Success? symposium, Washington, DC, June 11, 2006.

page 105 "In treatment guidelines known as . . . " Scott M. Grundy, James I. Cleeman, C. Noel Bairey Merz, H. Bryan Brewer, Luther T. Clark, Donald B. Hunninghake, Richard C. Pasternak, Sidney C. Smith, and Neil J. Stone, "Implications of Recent Clinical Trials for the National Cholesterol Education Program Adult Treatment Panel III Guidelines," *Journal of the American College of Cardiology* 44(2004): 720–732. Also see Scott M. Grundy, James I. Cleeman, Stephen R. Daniels, Karen A. Donato, Robert H. Eckel, Barry A. Franklin, David J. Gordon, et al., "Diagnosis and Management of the Metabolic Syndrome: An American Heart Association/National Heart, Lung, and Blood Institute Scientific Statement," *Circulation* 112(2005): 2735–2752.

page 106 "In 2003, Richard Kahn, . . . " Richard Kahn, John Buse, Ele Ferrannini, and Michael Stern, "The Metabolic Syndrome: Time for a Critical Appraisal: Joint Statement from the American Diabetes Association and the European Association for the Study of Diabetes," *Diabetologia* 48(2005): 1684–1699.

page 108 "One estimate suggests that . . . " Robert M. Kaplan, Theodore G. Ganiats, and Dominick L. Frosch, "Diagnostic and Treatment Decisions in US Healthcare," *Journal of Health Psychology* 9(2004): 29–40.

page 113 "A 2008 study of smokers . . . " Jane Ogden and Louisa Hills, "Understanding Sustained Behavior Change: The Role of Life Crises and the Process of Reinvention," *Health* 12(2008): 419–437.

page 114 "Patients on statins were the worst, . . . " J. A. Cramer, Á. Benedict, N. Muszbek, A. Keskinaslan, and Z. M. Khan, "The Significance of Compliance and Persistence in the Treatment of Diabetes, Hypertension and Dyslipidaemia: A Review," *International Journal of Clinical Practice* 62(2008): 76–87.

Chapter 6

page 116 "The test screened for phenylketonuria, . . . " Diane B. Paul, "Appendix 5: The History of Newborn Phenylketonuria Screening in the U.S.,"

Promoting Safe and Effective Genetic Testing in the United States, Final Report of the Task Force on Genetic Testing, September 1997.

page 117 "The US Preventive Services Task Force, . . . " The USPSTF is greatly underutilized by Americans; few outside the worlds of medicine and public health know it exists. But its Web site, www.ahrq.gov/CLINIC/uspstfix. htm, offers a thorough explanation for laypeople of which screening tests are recommended, which are not, and why.

page 118 "Even for a common disease like breast cancer, . . . " Joann G. Elmore, Mary B. Barton, Victoria M. Moceri, Sarah Polk, Philip J. Arena, and Suzanne W. Fletcher, "Ten-Year Risk of False Positive Screening Mammograms and Clinical Breast Examinations," *New England Journal of Medicine* 338(1998): 1089–1096.

page 120 "Take breast cancer, for example, . . . " Debbie Saslow, Carla Boetes, Sylie Burke, Steven Harms, Martin O. Leach, Constance D. Lehman, Elizabeth Morris, et al., "American Cancer Society Guidelines for Breast Screening with MRI as an Adjunct to Mammography," *CA: A Cancer Journal for Clinicians* 57(2007): 75–89.

page 122 "Andreas Vesalius was only 23 years old . . . " Daniel Garrison and Malcolm Hast, "*On the Fabric of the Human Body:* An Annotated Translation of the 1543 and 1555 Editions of Andreas Vesalius' *De Humani Corporis Fabrica,*" March 19, 2003, Northwestern University. http://vesalius. northwestern.edu/flash.html.

page 125 "One day in 1967 . . . " Godfrey N. Hounsfield, "Autobiography," in *The Nobel Prizes 1979,* Wilhelm Odelberg, ed. (Stockholm: Nobel Foundation, 1980). Also see Caroline Richmond, "Obituary: Sir Godfrey Hounsfield," *BMJ* 329(2004): 687.

page 125 "As Shannon Brownlee wrote . . . " Shannon Brownlee, *Overtreated: Why Too Much Medicine Is Making Us Sicker and Poorer* (New York: Bloomsbury, 2007).

page 126 "But the price arrow points . . . " Wayne T. Stockburger, "CT Imaging, Then and Now," *Radiology Management* 26(2004): 20–27.

pages 127–128 "Doctors in the United States ordered . . . " United States Government Accountability Office, *Medicare Part B Imaging Services: Rapid Spending Growth and Shift to Physician Offices Indicate Need for CMS to Consider Additional Management Practices,* GAO-08-452 (Washington, DC: Government Accounting Office, June 2008).

page 128 "Sales of imaging equipment . . . " Amy Brock, *Medical Imaging: Equipment and Related Products,* BCC Report HLC020E (Wellesley, MA: BCC Research, October 2007).

page 128 "Diagnostic radiology is routinely . . . " American Medical Group Association, "2008 Physician Compensation Survey," n.d. www. cejkasearch.com/compensation/amga_physician_compensation_survey. htm. Also see Radiological Society of North America, "Diagnostic Radiology Earns Highest Four-Year Pay Increase," *RSNA News,* October

2004. www.rsna.org/publications/rsnanews/oct04/salary-1.html.

page 128 "Clayton Christensen, DBA, a professor . . . " Mark D. Smith, "Disruptive Innovation: Can Health Care Learn from Other Industries? A Conversation with Clayton M. Christensen," *Health Affairs* 26(2007): w288–w295. For Christensen's exhaustive take on the health care system, see his recent book, *The Innovator's Prescription: A Disruptive Solution for Health Care* (New York: McGraw-Hill, 2009).

page 129 "In the mid-1990s, the International . . . " Claudia I. Henschke, David F. Yankelevitz, Daniel M. Libby, Mark W. Pasmantier, James P. Smith, and Olli S. Miettinen, "Survival of Patients with Stage I Lung Cancer Detected on CT Screening," *New England Journal of Medicine* 355(2006): 1763–1771.

page 130 "Dr. Bach had strong enough doubts . . . " Peter B. Bach, "Is Our Natural-History Model of Lung Cancer Wrong?" *Lancet Oncology* 9(2008): 693–697. See also Peter B. Bach, James R. Jett, Ugo Pastorino, Melvyn S. Tockman, Stephen J. Swensen, and Colin B. Begg, "Computed Tomography Screening and Lung Cancer Outcomes," *JAMA* 297(2007): 953–961.

page 131 "As for Dr. Henschke, . . . " Paul Goldberg, "Tobacco Company Liggett Gave $3.6 Million to Henschke for CT Screening Research," *The Cancer Letter*, March 25, 2008.

page 132 "'The first observation of cancer cells . . . '" The quote is from *Cancer Warrior: Accidental Discoveries: Part 2,* n.d. www.pbs.org/wgbh/nova/cancer/discoveries2.html. Papanicolaou's first paper on the test was George N. Papanicolaou and Herbert F. Traut, "The Diagnostic Value of Vaginal Smears in Carcinoma of the Uterus," *American Journal of Obstetrics and Gynecology* 42(1941): 193–206. See also George Nicholas Papanicolaou, *Diagnosis of Uterine Cancer by the Vaginal Smear* (New York: The Commonwealth Fund, 1943).

page 133 "In early 2009, a team from the International Agency . . . " Rengaswamy Sankaranarayanan, Bhagwan M. Nene, Surendra S. Shastri, Kasturi Jayant, Richard Muwonge, Atul M. Budukh, Sanjay Hingmire, et al., "HPV Screening for Cervical Cancer in Rural India," *New England Journal of Medicine* 360(2009): 1385–1394.

page 137 "It wasn't until 1975, . . . " S. G. Pauker and J. P. Kassirer, "Therapeutic Decision Making: A Cost-Benefit Analysis," *New England Journal of Medicine* 293(1975): 229–234.

Chapter 7

page 146 "Billions of dollars have been spent . . . " Guy B. Faguet, *The War on Cancer: An Anatomy of Failure, a Blueprint for the Future* (New York: Springer, 2008).

page 152 "Traditionally biomarkers are used . . . " The literature is full of reports of specific biomarker discoveries, but some good overviews of the principles of biomarkers for cancer include David F. Ransohoff, "Developing Molecular Biomarkers for Cancer," *Science* 299(2003): 1679–1680. Also see Walter Willett, "Cancer Prevention and Early Detection," *Cancer Epidemiology Bio-markers and Prevention* 12(2003): 252S; and Lee Hartwell, David Mankoff, Amanda Paulovich, Scott Ramsey, and Elizabeth Swisher, "Cancer Biomarkers: A Systems Approach," *Nature Biotechnology* 24(2006): 905–908.

page 154 "Take the case of prolactin. . . . " Jason D. Thorpe, Xiaobo Duan, Robin Forrest, Kimberly Lowe, Lauren Brown, Elliot Segal, Brad Nelson, Garnet L. Anderson, Martin McIntosh, and Nicole Urban, "Effects of Blood Collection Conditions on Ovarian Cancer Serum Markers," *PLoS One* 2(2007): e1281. Other papers noting the complications of cancer biomarkers are A. M. Nick and A. K. Sood, "The ROC 'n' Role of the Multiplex Assay for Early Detection of Ovarian Cancer," *Nature Clinical Practice Oncology* 5(2008): 568–569; and Lisa M. Schwartz, Steven Woloshin, Floyd J. Fowler, and H. Gilbert Welch, "Enthusiasm for Cancer Screening in the United States," *JAMA* 291(2004): 71–78.

page 157 "Soon enough, Dr. Gambhir . . . " Amelie M. Lutz, Juergen K. Willmann, Frank V. Cochran, Pritha Ray, Sanjiv S. Gambhir, "Cancer Screening: A Mathematical Model Relating Secreted Blood Biomarker Levels to Tumor Sizes," *PLoS Medicine* 5(2008): e170.

page 160 "Take the role of fat . . . " Osama Hamdy, "The Role of Adipose Tissue as an Endocrine Gland," *Current Diabetes Reports* 5(2005): 317–319.

page 162 "The Canary Foundation has made 'normal' . . . " Canary Foundation, "Baseline Program," n.d. http://canaryfoundation.org/baseline.cfm.

page 163 "When President Barack Obama . . . " Will Dunham, "Obama Cancer Cure Vow Requires More Funds—Experts," Reuters, February 25, 2009. www.reuters.com/article/companyNewsAndPR/idUSN2548079320090225. Also see Elizabeth Landau, "Where's the Cure for Cancer?" CNN.com, March 3, 2009. www.cnn.com/2009/HEALTH/03/03/cure.cancer.obama/index.html.

Chapter 8

page 169 "In 1961, a young scientist . . . " The definitive and highly readable account of Dr. Folkman's work is Robert Cooke's *Dr. Folkman's War: Angiogenesis and the Struggle to Defeat Cancer* (New York: Random House, 2001).

page 170 "'We believe that [EntreMed] . . . '" Justin Gillis, "Can EntreMed Live Up to Its Research Promise?" *Washington Post*, May 11, 1998.

page 170 "A few weeks later, *New York Times* . . . " Gina Kolata, "Hope in the Lab: A Special Report; A Cautious Awe Greets Drugs That Eradicate Tumors in Mice," *New York Times*, May 3, 1998.

page 171 "For every million people . . . " Erica S. Spatz, Maureen E. Canavan, and Mayur M. Desai, "From Here to JUPITER: Identifying New Patients for Statin Therapy Using Data from the 1999–2004 National Health and Nutrition Examination Survey," *Circulation: Cardiovascular Quality and Outcomes* 2(2009): 41–48.

page 172 "As in real life, STAR*D . . . " A. John Rush, "STAR*D: What Have We Learned?" *American Journal of Psychiatry* 164(2007): 201–204. An exhaustive history and the full results of STAR*D are available at www.edc. pitt.edu/stard.

page 176 "From the industry's point of view, . . . " A thorough assessment of the new era of pharmaceutical research can be found at Lawton R. Burns, ed., *The Business of Healthcare Innovation* (Cambridge, UK: Cambridge University Press, 2005). For a view from the other side of the fence, try Marcia Angell's *The Truth About the Drug Companies: How They Deceive Us and What to Do About It* (New York: Random House, 2005).

page 179 "That was the premise behind . . . " S. G. Chrysant, "The ALLHAT Study: Results and Clinical Implications," *QJM* 96(2003): 771–773.

page 180 "Acetylsalicylic acid, as aspirin is . . . " A. S. Tarnawski and T. C. Caves, "Aspirin in the XXI Century: Its Major Clinical Impact, Novel Mechanisms of Action, and New Safer Formulations," *Gastroenterology* 127(2004): 341–343.

page 181 "In May 2009, researchers from the University . . . " Alison H. Harrill, Paul B. Watkins, Stephen Su, Pamela K. Ross, David E. Harbourt, Ioannis M. Stylianou, Gary A. Boorman, et al., "Mouse Population-Guided Resequencing Reveals That Variants in *CD44* Contribute to Acetaminophen-Induced Liver Injury in Humans," *Genome Research,* May 5, 2009 [Epub ahead of print].

page 182 "Gleevec is remarkably effective . . . " Leslie A. Pray, "Gleevec: The Breakthrough in Cancer Treatment," *Nature Education* 1(2008). www.nature.com/ scitable/topicpage/Gleevec-the-Breakthrough-in-Cancer-Treatment-565.

page 182 "The standout example here is warfarin, . . . " International Warfarin Pharmacogenetics Consortium, "Estimation of the Warfarin Dose with Clinical and Pharmacogenetic Data," *New England Journal of Medicine* 360(2009): 753–764.

page 183 "Perhaps the best model here is Adjuvant!, . . . " The tool can be viewed at www.adjuvantonline.com. Details here come from Eric T. Rosenthal, "Adjuvant! Online Risk-Benefit Profiler: Assessing the Pros and Cons of Letting Patients Have Direct Access," *Oncology Times* 29(2007): 10–15. More recent related data are at Yu Shen, Wenli Dong, Barry W. Feig, Peter Ravdin, Richard L. Theriault, and Sharon H. Giordano, "Patterns of Treatment for Early Stage Breast Cancers at the M. D. Anderson Cancer Center from 1997 to 2004," *Cancer* 115(2009): 2041–2051.

page 185 "Within days, James Watson, . . . " James D. Watson, letter to the editor, *New York Times,* May 7, 1998.

page 187 "As of 2009, the company was testing Avastin . . . " Genentech, "Avastin: Development Pipeline," July 2009.

page 189 "In 2008, the *New York Times* ran another . . . " Gina Kolata and Andrew Pollack, "Costly Cancer Drug Offers Hope, but Also a Dilemma," *New York Times,* July 6, 2008.

Chapter 9

page 194 "Despite the emphasis in medicine . . . " For an eloquent explanation of the poorly understood art of prognosis, see Nicholas A. Christakis, *Death Foretold:*

Prophecy and Prognosis in Medical Care (Chicago: University of Chicago, 2001).

page 194 "In a classic 1982 study ... " D. M. Eddy, "Probabilistic Reasoning in Clinical Medicine: Problems and Opportunities," in *Judgment Under Uncertainty: Heuristics and Biases,* Daniel Kahneman, Paul Slovic, and Amos Tversky, eds. (New York: Cambridge University Press, 1982).

page 195 "'Because we do not know ... '" Alan Schwartz and George Bergus, *Medical Decision Making: A Physician's Guide* (Cambridge, UK: Cambridge University Press, 2008): 76.

page 196 "Not that uncertainty ... " The classic work on uncertainty was edited by the twin pillars of decision science, Daniel Kahneman and Amos Tversky, along with Paul Slovic, *Judgment Under Uncertainty: Heuristics and Biases* (New York: Cambridge University Press, 1982). Equally influential on my thinking here is Reid Hastie, *Rational Choice in an Uncertain World: The Psychology of Judgment and Decision Making* (New York: Sage Publications, 2009): 326.

page 196 "In many ways, uncertainty ... " Matt T. Bianchi, Brian M. Alexander, and Sydney S. Cash, "Incorporating Uncertainty into Medical Decision Making: An Approach to Unexpected Test Results," *Medical Decision Making* 29(2009): 116–124.

page 197 "We *try* to wield control, ... " Ellen Langer, "The Illusion of Control," *Journal of Personality and Social Psychology* 32(1975): 311–328.

page 197 "It's worth reminding ourselves, ... " This notion of a "good" decision comes from Schwartz, *Medical Decision Making: A Physician's Guide,* p. 4.

page 198 "Of all the tricks, techniques, ... " Benjamin Franklin, *The Writings of Benjamin Franklin, Volume III,* London, 1757–1775.

page 199 "The wisdom of Franklin's approach ... " C. O. Archer and D. Swearingen, "Application of Benjamin Franklin's Decision-Making Model to the Clinical Setting," *Nursing Forum* 16(1977): 319–328.

page 201 "Dr. Ornish has had particular ... " Dean Ornish, Jue Lin, Jennifer Daubenmier, Gerdi Weidner, Elissa Epel, Colleen Kemp, Mark Jesus M. Magbanua, et al., "Increased Telomerase Activity and Comprehensive Lifestyle Changes: A Pilot Study," *Lancet Oncology* 9(2008): 1048–1057. Also see Dean Ornish, Mark Jesus M. Magbanua, Gerdi Weidner, Vivian Weinberg, Colleen Kemp, Christopher Green, Michael D. Mattie, et al., "Changes in Prostate Gene Expression in Men Undergoing an Intensive Nutrition and Lifestyle Intervention," *Proceedings of the National Academy of Sciences of the United States of America* 105(2008): 8369–8374.

page 202 "This was the question that Eric Horvitz ... " Ryen White and Eric Horvitz, "Cyberchondria: Studies of the Escalation of Medical Concerns in Web Search," Microsoft Research, November 1, 2008.

page 205 "In a survey of about 500 ... " The quiz was first posed by David J. Malenka, John A. Baron, Sarah Johansen, Jon W. Wahrenberger, and Jonathan M. Ross in "The Framing Effect of Relative and Absolute Risk," *Journal of General Internal Medicine* 8(1993): 543–548.

page 205 "Now consider this survey, . . . " Dennis J. Mazur and David H. Hickam, "Treatment Preferences of Patients and Physicians: Influences of Summary Data When Framing Effects Are Controlled," *Medical Decision Making* 10(1990): 2–5.

page 207 "By and large, people are also prone . . . " Neil D. Weinstein and Elizabeth Lachendro, "Egocentrism as a Source of Unrealistic Optimism," *Personality and Social Psychology Bulletin* 8(1982): 195–200.

page 208 "Dr. Reyna called her observation . . . " Valerie F. Reyna, "A Theory of Medical Decision Making and Health: Fuzzy Trace Theory," *Medical Decision Making* 28(2008): 850–865. Also see her "Theories of Medical Decision Making and Health: An Evidence-Based Approach," *Medical Decision Making* 28(2008): 829–833.

page 209 "As Jerome Groopman, . . . " Jerome Groopman, *How Doctors Think* (Boston: Houghton Mifflin, 2007).

page 210 "As a 2008 paper in the journal *Medical Decision Making* . . . " Bonnie Spring, "Health Decision Making: Lynchpin of Evidence-Based Practice," *Medical Decision Making* 28(2008): 866–874.

page 212 "(Physicians have their own decision tools . . . " Amit X. Garg, Neill K. J. Adhikari, Heather McDonald, M. Patricia Rosas-Arellano, P. J. Devereaux, Joseph Beyene, Justina Sam, and R. Brian Haynes, "Effects of Computerized Clinical Decision Support Systems on Practitioner Performance and Patient Outcomes: A Systematic Review," *JAMA* 293(2005): 1223–1238.

page 212 "To answer that question, Dr. O'Connor . . . " A. M. O'Connor, D. Stacey, V. Entwistle, H. Llewellyn-Thomas, D. Rovner, M. Holmes-Rovner, V. Tait, J. Tetroe, V. Fiset, M. Barry, and J. Jones, "Decision Aids for People Facing Health Treatment or Screening Decisions," *Cochrane Database of Systematic Reviews Online*, no. 2 (2003): CD001431.

page 213 "Researchers at the Mayo Clinic . . . " Audrey J. Weymiller, Victor M. Montori, Lesley A. Jones, Amiram Gafni, Gordon H. Guyatt, Sandra C. Bryant, Teresa J. H. Christianson, Rebecca J. Mullan, and Steven A. Smith, "Helping Patients with Type 2 Diabetes Mellitus Make Treatment Decisions: Statin Choice Randomized Trial," *Archives of Internal Medicine* 167(2007): 1076–1082.

Chapter 10

pages 217–218 "Muscle weakness is a hallmark . . . " National Multiple Sclerosis Society, "About MS: Who Gets MS?" n.d. www.nationalmssociety.org/about-multiple-sclerosis/who-gets-ms/index.aspx.

page 224 "The shame of disease, . . . " Susan Sontag, *Illness as Metaphor* (New York: Farrar Straus and Giroux, 1978).

page 226 "The truly subversive notice . . . " PatientsLikeMe.com, "Our Philosophy: Openness Is a Good Thing," n.d. www.patientslikeme.com/about/openness.

page 226 "In 1990, Alan Westin, . . . " A. Westin, *Harris-Equifax Consumer Privacy Survey*, technical report, 1991. For a complete rundown of Westin's work and the slight variations in consumer preferences over time, see Pon-nurangam Kumaraguru and Lorrie Faith Cranor, *Privacy Indexes: A Survey of Westin's Studies,* CMU-ISRI-05-138, Institute for Software Research International, December 2005.

page 228 "With the pioneer spirit . . . " My discussion of the health seekers was informed by Sheila M. Rothman's wonderfully researched and deeply informed book *Living in the Shadow of Death: Tuberculosis and the Social Experience of Illness in American History* (Baltimore: Johns Hopkins University Press, 1995).

page 238 "In 2001, the American Medical Association . . . " This press release was dug up by Susannah Fox of the Pew Internet and American Life Project, and it was part of her presentation at a Health 2.0 conference in March 2008. http://e-patients.net/archives/2008/03/flashback-to-2001.html.

Coda

page 243 "As patients typed in the answers . . . " Warner Slack's work was introduced to me by Jason Bobe at the Personal Genome Project. W. V. Slack, "Patient Power: A Patient-Oriented Value System," in *Computer Diagnosis and Diagnostic Methods: Proceedings of the Second Conference on the Diagnostic Process,* John A. Jacquez, ed. (Springfield, IL: Charles C. Thomas, 1972).

page 244 "They were trained to say . . . " Warner V. Slack, "A 67-Year-Old Man Who E-Mails His Physician," *JAMA* 292(2004): 2255–2261; and W. Slack, "Cybermedicine for the Patient," *American Journal of Preventive Medicine* 32(2007): S135–S136.

page 244 "Even 30 years later, in 1991, . . . " B. Fisher and N. Britten, "Patient Access to Records: Expectations of Hospital Doctors and Experiences of Cancer Patients," *British Journal of General Practice* 43(1993): 52–56.

page 245 "A 2007 survey of primary care . . . " Giridhar Mallya, Craig Evan Pollack, and Daniel Polsky, "Are Primary Care Physicians Ready to Practice in a Consumer-Driven Environment?" *American Journal of Managed Care* 14(2008): 661–668.

page 247 "'We've got a health care delivery system . . . '" Mark McLellan, remarks delivered at the Patient-Centric Leadership Forum, Center for Medicine in the Public Interest, August 1, 2008.

page 249 "In part, I take my cue . . . " Donald M. Berwick, "What 'Patient-Centered' Should Mean: Confessions of an Extremist," *Health Affairs* 28(2009): w555–w565.

page 250 "These fees do, in fact, . . . " Lance C. Goudzwaard, "Point-of-Service Collections in Healthcare," Surgistrategies.com, September 1, 2007. www.vpico.com/articlemanager/printerfriendly.aspx?article=153461.

page 250 "As Shannon Brownlee demonstrated . . . " Shannon Brownlee, *Overtreated: Why Too Much Medicine Is Making Us Sicker and Poorer* (New York: Bloomsbury, 2008); and Atul Gawande, "The Cost Conundrum," *New Yorker,* June 1, 2009.

Bibliography

Al-Shahi Salman, R., W. N. Whiteley, and C. Warlow. "Screening Using Whole-Body Magnetic Resonance Imaging Scanning: Who Wants an Incidentaloma?" *J Med Screen* 14(2007): 2–4.

Alemany, M., J. A. Fernandez-Lopez, A. Petrobelli, M. Granada, M. Foz, and X. Remesar. "[Weight Loss in a Patient with Morbid Obesity Under Treatment with Oleoyl-Estrone]." *Med Clin (Barc)* 121(2003): 496–99.

Ancker, J. S., and D. Kaufman. "Rethinking Health Numeracy: A Multidisciplinary Literature Review." *J Am Med Inform Assoc* 14(2007): 713–21.

Archer, C. O., and D. Swearingen. "Application of Benjamin Franklin's Decision-Making Model to the Clinical Setting." *Nurs Forum* 16(1977): 319–28.

Arias, E. "United States Life Tables, 2004." *Natl Vital Stat Rep* 56(2007): 1–39.

Austin, H. "An Epidemic Averted through Medical Screening." *J Med Screen* 12(2005): 1–2.

Bach, P. B. "Is Our Natural-History Model of Lung Cancer Wrong?" *Lancet Oncol* 9(2008): 693–97.

Bach, P. B., J. R. Jett, U. Pastorino, M. S. Tockman, S. J. Swensen, and C. B. Begg. "Computed Tomography Screening and Lung Cancer Outcomes." *JAMA* 297(2007): 953–61.

Bader, P., P. McDonald, and P. Selby. "An Algorithm for Tailoring Pharmacotherapy for Smoking Cessation: Results from a Delphi Panel of International Experts." *Tob Control* 18(2009): 34–42.

Baker, L. C., S. W. Atlas, and C. C. Afendulis. "Expanded Use of Imaging Technology and the Challenge of Measuring Value." *Health Aff (Millwood)* 27(2008): 1467–78.

Bandura, A. "Self-Efficacy: Toward a Unifying Theory of Behavioral Change." *Psychol Rev* 84(1977): 191–215.

Bandura, A., D. Ross, and S. A. Ross. "Transmission of Aggression through Imitation of Aggressive Models." *J Abnorm Soc Psychol* 63(1961): 575–82.

Barry, M. J. "Screening for Prostate Cancer—The Controversy That Refuses to Die." *N Engl J Med* 360(2009): 1351–54.

Bellg, A. J., B. Borrelli, B. Resnick, J. Hecht, D. S. Minicucci, M. Ory, G. Ogedegbe, D. Orwig, D. Ernst, and S. Czajkowski. "Enhancing Treatment

Fidelity in Health Behavior Change Studies: Best Practices and Recommendations from the NIH Behavior Change Consortium." *Health Psychol* 23(2004): 443–51.

Berrington de Gonzalez, A. "Computed Tomography Screening: Safe and Effective?" *J Med Screen* 14(2007): 165–68.

Berry, D. A. "The Screening Mammography Paradox: Better When Found, Perhaps Better Not to Find." *Br J Cancer* 98(2008): 1729–30.

Berwick, D. M. "Disseminating Innovations in Health Care." *JAMA* 289(2003): 1969–75.

Bianchi, M. T., B. M. Alexander, and S. S. Cash. "Incorporating Uncertainty into Medical Decision Making: An Approach to Unexpected Test Results." *Med Decis Making* 29(2009): 116–24.

Black, W. C., and H. G. Welch. "Screening for Disease." *AJR Am J Roentgenol* 168(1997): 3–11.

Brownlee, S. *Overtreated: Why Too Much Medicine Is Making Us Sicker and Poorer.* New York: Bloomsbury, 2008.

Bruenn, H. G. "Clinical Notes on the Illness and Death of President Franklin D. Roosevelt." *Ann Intern Med* 72(1970): 579–91.

Buchannan, A. *From Chance to Choice: Genetics and Justice.* Cambridge, UK: Cambridge University Press, 2001.

Buetow, K. H. "Cyberinfrastructure: Empowering a 'Third Way' in Biomedical Research." *Science* 308(2005): 821–24.

Burger, I. M., and N. E. Kass. "Screening in the Dark: Ethical Considerations of Providing Screening Tests to Individuals When Evidence Is Insufficient to Support Screening Populations." *Am J Bioeth* 9(2009): 3–14.

Burns, L. R. *The Business of Healthcare Innovation.* Cambridge, UK: Cambridge University Press, 2005.

Cameron, A. J., J. E. Shaw, and P. Z. Zimmet. "The Metabolic Syndrome: Prevalence in Worldwide Populations." *Endocrinol Metab Clin North Am* 33(2004): 351–75.

Canary Foundation. "Canary Foundation—Baseline Program." n.d. canaryfoundation.org/baseline.cfm.

Canick, J. "Safety First: Choices in Antenatal Screening for Down's Syndrome." *J Med Screen* 10(2003): 55.

Cassidy, M. R., J. S. Roberts, T. D. Bird, E. J. Steinbart, L. A. Cupples, C. A. Chen, E. Linnenbringer, and R. C. Green. "Comparing Test-Specific Distress of Susceptibility versus Deterministic Genetic Testing for Alzheimer's Disease." *Alzheimers Dement* 4(2008): 406–13.

Chan, D. C., P. A. Heidenreich, M. C. Weinstein, and G. C. Fonarow. "Heart Failure Disease Management Programs: A Cost-Effectiveness Analysis." *Am Heart J* 155(2008): 332–38.

Chao, S., J. S. Roberts, T. M. Marteau, R. Silliman, L. A. Cupples, and R. C. Green. "Health Behavior Changes after Genetic Risk Assessment for

Alzheimer Disease: The REVEAL Study." *Alzheimer Dis Assoc Disord* 22(2008): 94–97.

Charles, C., A. Gafni, and T. Whelan. "Decision-Making in the Physician-Patient Encounter: Revisiting the Shared Treatment Decision-Making Model." *Soc Sci Med* 49(1999): 651–61.

Chaudhry, B., J. Wang, S. Wu, M. Maglione, W. Mojica, E. Roth, S. C. Morton, and P. G. Shekelle. "Systematic Review: Impact of Health Information Technology on Quality, Efficiency, and Costs of Medical Care." *Ann Intern Med* 144(2006): 742–52.

Christakis, N. A. *Death Foretold Prophecy and Prognosis in Medical Care.* New York: University of Chicago, 2001.

Christakis, N. A., and J. H. Fowler. *Connected: The Surprising Power of Our Social Networks and How They Shape Our Lives.* New York: Little, Brown, 2009.

———. "The Spread of Obesity in a Large Social Network over 32 Years." *N Engl J Med* 357(2007): 370–79.

———. "The Collective Dynamics of Smoking in a Large Social Network." *N Engl J Med* 358(2008): 2249–58.

Christensen, C. *The Innovator's Prescription: A Disruptive Solution for Health Care.* New York: McGraw-Hill, 2008.

Chrysant, S. G. "The ALLHAT Study: Results and Clinical Implications." *QJM* 96(2003): 771–73.

Church, G. M. "From Systems Biology to Synthetic Biology." *Mol Syst Biol* 1(2005): 2005.0032.

Clemens, C. J., S. A. Davis, and A. R. Bailey. "The False-Positive in Universal Newborn Hearing Screening." *Pediatrics* 106(2000): E7.

Collins, V. R., E. E. Muggli, M. Riley, S. Palma, and J. L. Halliday. "Is Down Syndrome a Disappearing Birth Defect?" *J Pediatr* 152(2008): 20–24.

Cooke, R. *Dr. Folkman's War: Angiogenesis and the Struggle to Defeat Cancer.* New York: Random House, 2001.

Couzin, J. "Drug Safety: Gaps in the Safety Net." *Science* 307(2005): 196–98.

Cramer, J. A., A. Benedict, N. Muszbek, A. Keskinaslan, and Z. M. Khan. "The Significance of Compliance and Persistence in the Treatment of Diabetes, Hypertension and Dyslipidaemia: A Review." *Int J Clin Pract* 62(2008): 76–87.

de Nooijer, J., L. Lechner, M. Candel, and H. de Vries. "A Randomized Controlled Study of Short-Term and Long-Term Effects of Tailored Information Versus General Information on Intention and Behavior Related to Early Detection of Cancer." *Cancer Epidemiol Biomarkers Prev* 11(2002): 1489–91.

DeMonaco, H. J., and E. von Hippel. "Reducing Medical Costs and Improving Quality Via Self-Management Tools." *PLoS Med* 4(2007): e104.

DiClemente, C. C., A. S. Marinilli, M. Singh, and L. E. Bellino. "The Role of

Feedback in the Process of Health Behavior Change." *Am J Health Behav* 25(2001): 217–27.

Dobbin, K. K., D. G. Beer, M. Meyerson, T. J. Yeatman, W. L. Gerald, J. W. Jacobson, B. Conley, K. H. Buetow, M. Heiskanen, R. M. Simon, J. D. Minna, L. Girard, D. E. Misek, J. M. Taylor, S. Hanash, K. Naoki, D. N. Hayes, C. Ladd-Acosta, S. A. Enkemann, A. Viale, and T. J. Giordano. "Interlaboratory Comparability Study of Cancer Gene Expression Analysis Using Oligonucleotide Microarrays." *Clin Cancer Res* 11(2005): 565–72.

Dunham, W. "Obama Cancer Cure Vow Requires More Funds: Experts." Reuters www.reuters.com/article/companyNewsAndPR/idUSN2548079320090225.

Eckmanns, T., J. Bessert, M. Behnke, P. Gastmeier, and H. Ruden. "Compliance with Antiseptic Hand Rub Use in Intensive Care Units: The Hawthorne Effect." *Infect Control Hosp Epidemiol* 27(2006): 931–34.

Eddy, D. M., and L. Schlessinger. "Archimedes: A Trial-Validated Model of Diabetes." *Diabetes Care* 26(2003): 3093–101.

———. "Validation of the Archimedes Diabetes Model." *Diabetes Care* 26(2003): 3102–10.

Egan, J. F., P. A. Benn, C. M. Zelop, A. Bolnick, E. Gianferrari, and A. F. Borgida. "Down Syndrome Births in the United States from 1989 to 2001." *Am J Obstet Gynecol* 191(2004): 1044–48.

Elstein, A. S., and A. Schwartz. "Clinical Problem Solving and Diagnostic Decision Making: Selective Review of the Cognitive Literature." *BMJ* 324(2002): 729–32.

Erkanli, A., D. D. Taylor, D. Dean, F. Eksir, D. Egger, J. Geyer, B. H. Nelson, B. Stone, H. A. Fritsche, and R. B. Roden. "Application of Bayesian Modeling of Autologous Antibody Responses against Ovarian Tumor-Associated Antigens to Cancer Detection." *Cancer Res* 66(2006): 1792–98.

Evans, J. P., and W. Burke. "Genetic Exceptionalism. Too Much of a Good Thing?" *Genet Med* 10(2008): 500–501.

Faguet, G. *The War on Cancer: An Anatomy of Failure, a Blueprint for the Future*. Dordrecht, The Netherlands: Springer, 2009.

Feil, P. H., J. S. Grauer, C. C. Gadbury-Amyot, K. Kula, and M. D. McCunniff. "Intentional Use of the Hawthorne Effect to Improve Oral Hygiene Compliance in Orthodontic Patients." *J Dent Educ* 66(2002): 1129–35.

Fletcher, R. H. "Colorectal Cancer Screening on Stronger Footing." *N Engl J Med* 359(2008): 1285–87.

Fletcher, S. W., and G. A. Colditz. "Failure of Estrogen Plus Progestin Therapy for Prevention." *JAMA* 288(2002): 366–68.

Fowler, J. H., and N. A. Christakis. "Dynamic Spread of Happiness in a Large Social Network: Longitudinal Analysis over 20 Years in the Framingham Heart Study." *BMJ* 337(2008): a2338.

Fowler, J. H., C. T. Dawes, and N. A. Christakis. "Model of Genetic Variation in Human Social Networks." *Proc Natl Acad Sci USA* 106(2009): 1720–24.

Franklin, B. *The Writings of Benjamin Franklin, Volume III,* London, 1757–1775.

Frantz, S. "Drug Discovery: Playing Dirty." *Nature* 437(2005): 942–43.

Gale, E. A. "The Myth of the Metabolic Syndrome." *Diabetologia* 48(2005): 1679–83.

Garattini, S., and I. Chalmers. "Patients and the Public Deserve Big Changes in Evaluation of Drugs." *BMJ* 338(2009): b1025.

Gardiner, C., I. Longair, M. A. Pescott, H. Erwin, J. Hills, S. J. Machin, and H. Cohen. "Self-Monitoring of Oral Anticoagulation: Does It Work Outside Trial Conditions?" *J Clin Pathol* 62(2009): 168–171.

Garg, A. X., N. K. Adhikari, H. McDonald, M. P. Rosas-Arellano, P. J. Devereaux, J. Beyene, J. Sam, and R. B. Haynes. "Effects of Computerized Clinical Decision Support Systems on Practitioner Performance and Patient Outcomes: A Systematic Review." *JAMA* 293(2005): 1223–38.

Garrison, D., and M. Hast. *On the Fabric of the Human Body:* An Annotated Translation of the 1543 and 1555 Editions of Andreas Vesalius' *De Humani Corporis Fabrica.* March 19, 2003. Northwestern University. vesalius. northwestern.edu/flash.html.

Gattellari, M., K. J. Voigt, P. N. Butow, and M. H. Tattersall. "When the Treatment Goal Is Not Cure: Are Cancer Patients Equipped to Make Informed Decisions?" *J Clin Oncol* 20(2002): 503–513.

Gelenberg, A. J., M. E. Thase, R. E. Meyer, F. K. Goodwin, M. M. Katz, H. C. Kraemer, W. Z. Potter, R. C. Shelton, M. Fava, A. Khan, M. H. Trivedi, P. T. Ninan, J. J. Mann, S. Bergeson, J. Endicott, J. H. Kocsis, A. C. Leon, H. K. Manji, and J. F. Rosenbaum. "The History and Current State of Antidepressant Clinical Trial Design: A Call to Action for Proof-of-Concept Studies." *J Clin Psychiatry* 69(2008): 1513–28.

Gigerenzer, G. *Calculated Risks: How to Know When Numbers Deceive You.* New York: Simon and Schuster, 2003.

Gollust S. E., S. C. Hull, and B. S. Wilfond. "Limitations of Direct-to-Consumer Advertising for Clinical Genetic Testing." *JAMA* 288(2002): 1762–67.

Green, M. J., and J. R. Botkin. "'Genetic Exceptionalism' in Medicine: Clarifying the Differences between Genetic and Nongenetic Tests." *Ann Intern Med* 138(2003): 571–75.

Greene, J. *Prescribing by Numbers: Drugs and the Definition of Disease.* Baltimore: Johns Hopkins University Press, 2008.

Grimes, D. A., and K. F. Schulz. "Uses and Abuses of Screening Tests." *Lancet* 359(2002): 881–84.

Groopman, J. *How Doctors Think.* Boston: Houghton Mifflin, 2007.

Grundy, S. M. "Drug Therapy of the Metabolic Syndrome: Minimizing the Emerging Crisis in Polypharmacy." *Nat Rev Drug Discov* 5(2006): 295–309.

Grundy, S. M., J. I. Cleeman, S. R. Daniels, K. A. Donato, R. H. Eckel, B. A.

Franklin, D. J. Gordon, R. M. Krauss, P. J. Savage, S. C. Smith, J. A. Spertus, and F. Costa. "Diagnosis and Management of the Metabolic Syndrome: An American Heart Association/National Heart, Lung, and Blood Institute Scientific Statement." *Circulation* 112(2005): 2735–52.

Gwyn, K., S. W. Vernon, and P. M. Conoley. "Intention to Pursue Genetic Testing for Breast Cancer among Women Due for Screening Mammography." *Cancer Epidemiol Biomarkers Prev* 12(2003): 96–102.

Hamdy, O. "The Role of Adipose Tissue as an Endocrine Gland." *Curr Diab Rep* 5(2005): 317–19.

Handelsman, Y. "Guest Editorial." *Metab Syndr Relat Disord* 3(2005): 281–83.

Hardy, J., and A. Singleton. "Genomewide Association Studies and Human Disease." *N Engl J Med* 360(2009): 1759–68.

Hartwell, L., D. Mankoff, A. Paulovich, S. Ramsey, and E. Swisher. "Cancer Biomarkers: A Systems Approach." *Nat Biotechnol* 24(2006): 905–908.

Hastie, R. *Rational Choice in an Uncertain World: The Psychology of Judgment and Decision Making.* New York: Sage, 2009.

Helfand, M. "Shared Decision Making, Decision Aids, and Risk Communication." *Med Decis Making* 27(2007): 516–17.

Henschke, C. I., D. F. Yankelevitz, D. M. Libby, M. W. Pasmantier, J. P. Smith, and O. S. Miettinen. "Survival of Patients with Stage I Lung Cancer Detected on CT Screening." *N Engl J Med* 355(2006): 1763–71.

Hersh, A. L., M. L. Stefanick, and R. S. Stafford. "National Use of Postmenopausal Hormone Therapy: Annual Trends and Response to Recent Evidence." *JAMA* 291(2004): 47–53.

Heshka, S., J. W. Anderson, R. L. Atkinson, F. L. Greenway, J. O. Hill, S. D. Phinney, R. L. Kolotkin, K. Miller-Kovach, and F. X. Pi-Sunyer. "Weight Loss with Self-Help Compared with a Structured Commercial Program: A Randomized Trial." *JAMA* 289(2003): 1792–98.

Hiraki, S., C. A. Chen, J. S. Roberts, L. A. Cupples, and R. C. Green. "Perceptions of Familial Risk in Those Seeking a Genetic Risk Assessment for Alzheimer's Disease." *J Genet Couns* 18(2009): 130–36.

Hirschhorn, J. N. "Genomewide Association Studies—Illuminating Biologic Pathways." *N Engl J Med* 360(2009): 1699–1701.

Hood, L., J. R. Heath, M. E. Phelps, and B. Lin. "Systems Biology and New Technologies Enable Predictive and Preventative Medicine." *Science* 306(2004): 640–43.

Hunter, D. J., M. J. Khoury, and J. M. Drazen. "Letting the Genome Out of the Bottle—Will We Get Our Wish?" *N Engl J Med* 358(2008): 105–107.

"The Imaging Boom." *Health Aff (Millwood)* 27(2008): 1466.

The International Warfarin Pharmacogenetics Consortium. "Estimation of the Warfarin Dose with Clinical and Pharmacogenetic Data." *N Eng J Med* 360(2009): 753–64.

Irving, C., A. Basu, S. Richmond, J. Burn, and C. Wren. "Twenty-Year Trends in Prevalence and Survival of Down Syndrome." *Eur J Hum Genet* 16(2008): 1336–40.

Jaffe, A. S., L. Babuin, and F. S. Apple. "Biomarkers in Acute Cardiac Disease: The Present and the Future." *J Am Coll Cardiol* 48(2006): 1–11.

Jolliffe, N., E. Maslansky, F. Rudensey, M. Simon, and A. Faulkner. "Dietary Control of Serum Cholesterol in Clinical Practice." *Circulation* 24(1961): 1415–21.

Kahn, R. "Dealing with Complexity in Clinical Diabetes: The Value of Archimedes." *Diabetes Care* 26(2003): 3168–71.

Kahn, R., J. Buse, E. Ferrannini, and M. Stern. "The Metabolic Syndrome: Time for a Critical Appraisal. Joint Statement from the American Diabetes Association and the European Association for the Study of Diabetes." *Diabetologia* 48(2005): 1684–99.

Kahneman, D. *Judgment Under Uncertainty: Heuristics and Biases.* New York: Cambridge University Press, 1982.

Kamerow, D. "Waiting for the Genetic Revolution." *BMJ* 336(2008): 22.

Kannel, W. B. "Risk Stratification in Hypertension: New Insights from the Framingham Study." *Am J Hypertens* 13(2000): 3S–10S.

Kassirer, J. *On the Take: How Medicine's Complicity with Big Business Can Endanger Your Health.* New York: Oxford University Press, 2005.

Katsanis, S. H., G. Javitt, and K. Hudson. "Public Health: A Case Study of Personalized Medicine." *Science* 320(2008): 53–54.

Kennedy, M. *A Brief History of Disease, Science and Medicine from the Ice Age to the Genome Project.* Cincinnati: Writer's Collective, 2004.

Khoury, M. J. "Genetics and Genomics in Practice: The Continuum from Genetic Disease to Genetic Information in Health and Disease." *Genet Med* 5(2003): 261–68.

Khoury, M. J., A. Berg, R. Coates, J. Evans, S. M. Teutsch, and L. A. Bradley. "The Evidence Dilemma in Genomic Medicine." *Health Aff (Millwood)* 27(2008): 1600–11.

Klein, R. D. "Gene Patents and Genetic Testing in the United States." *Nat Biotechnol* 25(2007): 989–90.

Klem, M. L., and R. C. Klesges. "Competition in a Minimal-Contact Weight-Loss Program." *J Consult Clin Psychol* 56(1988): 142–44.

Kraft, P., and D. J. Hunter. "Genetic Risk Prediction—Are We There Yet?" *N Engl J Med* 360(2009): 1701–1703.

Kraft, P., S. Wacholder, M. C. Cornelis, F. B. Hu, R. B. Hayes, G. Thomas, R. Hoover, D. J. Hunter, and S. Chanock. "Beyond Odds Ratios—Communicating Disease Risk Based on Genetic Profiles." *Nat Rev Genet* 10(2009): 264–69.

Kreuter, M. W., and V. J. Strecher. "Do Tailored Behavior Change Messages Enhance the Effectiveness of Health Risk Appraisal? Results from a Randomized Trial." *Health Educ Res* 11(1996): 97–105.

Kuller, L., J. Neaton, A. Caggiula, and L. Falvo-Gerard. "Primary Prevention of Heart Attacks: The Multiple Risk Factor Intervention Trial." *Am J Epidemiol* 112(1980): 185–99.

Landau, E. "Where's the Cure for Cancer?" CNN.com, March 3, 2009. www.cnn.com/2009/HEALTH/03/03/cure.cancer.obama/index.html.

Lane, K., and O. Boyd. "Computer Says 2.5 Litres—How Best to Incorporate Intelligent Software into Clinical Decision Making in the Intensive Care Unit?" *Crit Care* 13(2009): 111.

Langer, E. "The Illusion of Control." *J Pers Soc Psychol* 32(1975): 311–28.

Leape, L. L., and D. M. Berwick. "Five Years After to Err Is Human: What Have We Learned?" *JAMA* 293(2005): 2384–90.

Lee, T. H., and T. A. Brennan. "Direct-to-Consumer Marketing of High-Technology Screening Tests." *N Engl J Med* 346(2002): 529–31.

Lehrer, J. *How We Decide*. Boston: Houghton Mifflin Harcourt, 2009.

Lenfant, C. "Shattuck Lecture—Clinical Research to Clinical Practice—Lost in Translation?" *N Engl J Med* 349(2003): 868–74.

Leslie, E., A. L. Marshall, N. Owen, and A. Bauman. "Engagement and Retention of Participants in a Physical Activity Website." *Prev Med* 40(2005): 54–59.

Levitt, S. D., and J. A. List. "Was There Really a Hawthorne Effect at the Hawthorne Plant? An Analysis of the Original Illumination Experiments." National Bureau of Economic Research Working Paper No. 15016. May 2009.

Levy, A. G., and J. C. Hershey. "Value-Induced Bias in Medical Decision Making." *Med Decis Making* 28(2008): 269–76.

Levy, D. *Change of Heart: Unraveling the Mysteries of Cardiovascular Disease*. New York: Vintage, 2006.

Link, L. B., L. Robbins, C. A. Mancuso, and M. E. Charlson. "How Do Cancer Patients Who Try to Take Control of Their Disease Differ from Those Who Do Not?" *Eur J Cancer Care (Engl)* 13(2004): 219–26.

Lloyd, A. J. "The Extent of Patients' Understanding of the Risk of Treatments." *Qual Health Care* 10 Suppl 1 (2001): i14–i18.

Lundberg, G. D. "Low-Tech Autopsies in the Era of High-Tech Medicine: Continued Value for Quality Assurance and Patient Safety." *JAMA* 280(1998): 1273–74.

Lutz, A. M., J. K. Willmann, F. V. Cochran, P. Ray, and S. S. Gambhir. "Cancer Screening: A Mathematical Model Relating Secreted Blood Biomarker Levels to Tumor Sizes." *PLoS Med* 5(2008): e170.

Mahnken, J. D., W. Chan, D. H. Freeman, and J. L. Freeman. "Reducing the Effects of Lead-Time Bias, Length Bias and Over-Detection in Evaluating Screening Mammography: A Censored Bivariate Data Approach." *Stat Methods Med Res* 17(2008): 643–63.

Malenka, D. J., J. A. Baron, S. Johansen, J. W. Wahrenberger, and J. M. Ross. "The Framing Effect of Relative and Absolute Risk." *J Gen Intern Med* 8(1993): 543–48.

Marcia, A. *The Truth About the Drug Companies: How They Deceive Us and What to Do About It.* New York: Random House, 2005.

Marcus, B. H., B. C. Bock, B. M. Pinto, L. H. Forsyth, M. B. Roberts, and R. M. Traficante. "Efficacy of an Individualized, Motivationally-Tailored Physical Activity Intervention." *Ann Behav Med* 20(1998): 174–80.

Marmot, M. G. *The Status Syndrome: How Social Standing Affects Our Health and Longevity.* New York: Holt, 2005.

Marmot, M. G., G. D. Smith, S. Stansfeld, C. Patel, F. North, J. Head, I. White, E. Brunner, and A. Feeney. "Health Inequalities among British Civil Servants: The Whitehall II Study." *Lancet* 337(1991): 1387–93.

Mazur, D. J., and D. H. Hickam. "Treatment Preferences of Patients and Physicians: Influences of Summary Data When Framing Effects Are Controlled." *Med Decis Making* 10(1990): 2–5.

McGregor, M., J. A. Hanley, J. F. Boivin, and R. G. McLean. "Screening for Prostate Cancer: Estimating the Magnitude of Overdetection." *CMAJ* 159(1998): 1368–72.

McGuire, A. L., R. Fisher, P. Cusenza, K. Hudson, M. A. Rothstein, D. McGraw, S. Matteson, J. Glaser, and D. E. Henley. "Confidentiality, Privacy, and Security of Genetic and Genomic Test Information in Electronic Health Records: Points to Consider." *Genet Med* 10(2008): 495–99.

McNeil, B. J., and S. J. Adelstein. "Determining the Value of Diagnostic and Screening Tests." *J Nucl Med* 17(1976): 439–48.

"Medical Devices." *Health Aff (Millwood)* 27(2008): 1522.

Metropolis, N. "The Beginning of the Monte Carlo Method." *Los Alamos Sci* Special Issue (1987): 125–30.

Miyaki, K., A. Hara, M. Naito, T. Naito, and T. Nakayama. "Two New Criteria of the Metabolic Syndrome: Prevalence and the Association with Brachial-Ankle Pulse Wave Velocity in Japanese Male Workers." *J Occup Health* 48(2006): 134–40.

Morton, C. C., and W. E. Nance. "Newborn Hearing Screening—A Silent Revolution." *N Engl J Med* 354(2006): 2151–64.

Moser, M. "Historical Perspectives on the Management of Hypertension." *J Clin Hypertens (Greenwich)* 8 Suppl 2 (2006): 15–20.

Murphy, K. *Measuring the Gains from Medical Research: An Economic Approach.* New York: University of Chicago, 2003.

Murphy, K. M., and R. H. Topel. "The Value of Health and Longevity." *J Polit Econ* 114(2006): 871–904.

Murray, C. J., A. D. Lopez, J. T. Barofsky, C. Bryson-Cahn, and R. Lozano. "Estimating Population Cause-Specific Mortality Fractions from In-Hospital Mortality: Validation of a New Method." *PLoS Med* 4(2007): e326.

"My Genome. So What?" *Nature* 456(2008): 1.

Nagle, C., R. Hodges, R. Wolfe, and E. M. Wallace. "Reporting Down

Syndrome Screening Results: Women's Understanding of Risk." *Prenat Diagn* 29(2009): 234–39.

Naish, J. "Our Health, Our Care, Our Say." *J Med Screen* 13(2006): 56–57.

Nakar, S., S. Vinker, S. Neuman, E. Kitai, and J. Yaphe. "Baseline Tests or Screening: What Tests Do Family Physicians Order Routinely on Their Healthy Patients?" *J Med Screen* 9(2002): 133–34.

Nelson, N. J. "Virtual Colonoscopy Accepted as Primary Colon Cancer Screening Test." *J Natl Cancer Inst* 100(2008): 1492–99.

Neuman, H. B., M. E. Charlson, and L. K. Temple. "Is There a Role for Decision Aids in Cancer-Related Decisions?" *Crit Rev Oncol Hematol* 62(2007): 240–50.

Ng, P. C., Q. Zhao, S. Levy, R. L. Strausberg, and J. C. Venter. "Individual Genomes Instead of Race for Personalized Medicine." *Clin Pharmacol Ther* 84(2008): 306–309.

Nick, A. M., and A. K. Sood. "The ROC 'n' Role of the Multiplex Assay for Early Detection of Ovarian Cancer." *Nat Clin Pract Oncol* 5(2008): 568–69.

Nidetch, J. *The Story of Weight Watchers*. New York: Signet Books, 1970.

O'Connor, A. M., D. Stacey, V. Entwistle, H. Llewellyn-Thomas, D. Rovner, M. Holmes-Rovner, V. Tait, J. Tetroe, V. Fiset, M. Barry, and J. Jones. "Decision Aids for People Facing Health Treatment or Screening Decisions." *Cochrane Database Syst Rev* No. 2 (2003): CD001431.

O'Connor, A. M., J. E. Wennberg, F. Legare, H. A. Llewellyn-Thomas, B. W. Moulton, K. R. Sepucha, A. G. Sodano, and J. S. King. "Toward the 'Tipping Point': Decision Aids and Informed Patient Choice." *Health Aff (Millwood)* 26(2007): 716–25.

O'Malley, P. G., and A. J. Taylor. "Unregulated Direct-to-Consumer Marketing and Self-Referral for Screening Imaging Services: A Call to Action." *Arch Intern Med* 164(2004): 2406–2408.

Ogden, J., and L. Hills. "Understanding Sustained Behavior Change: The Role of Life Crises and the Process of Reinvention." *Health (London)* 12(2008): 419–37.

Olivotto, I. A., C. D. Bajdik, P. M. Ravdin, C. H. Speers, A. J. Coldman, B. D. Norris, G. J. Davis, S. K. Chia, and K. A. Gelmon. "Population-Based Validation of the Prognostic Model Adjuvant! for Early Breast Cancer." *J Clin Oncol* 23(2005): 2716–25.

Ornish, D., J. Lin, J. Daubenmier, G. Weidner, E. Epel, C. Kemp, M. J. Magbanua, R. Marlin, L. Yglecias, P. R. Carroll, and E. H. Blackburn. "Increased Telomerase Activity and Comprehensive Lifestyle Changes: A Pilot Study." *Lancet Oncol* 9(2008): 1048–57.

Ornish, D., M. J. Magbanua, G. Weidner, V. Weinberg, C. Kemp, C. Green, M. D. Mattie, R. Marlin, J. Simko, K. Shinohara, C. M. Haqq, and P. R. Carroll. "Changes in Prostate Gene Expression in Men Undergoing an

Intensive Nutrition and Lifestyle Intervention." *Proc Natl Acad Sci USA* 105(2008): 8369–74.

Paez, K. A., L. Zhao, and W. Hwang. "Rising Out-of-Pocket Spending for Chronic Conditions: A Ten-Year Trend." *Health Aff (Millwood)* 28(2009): 15–25.

Patnaik, M., M. J. Renda, M. C. Athanasiou, and C. R. Reed. "The Role of Pharmacogenetics in Treating Central Nervous System Disorders." *Exp Biol Med (Maywood)* 233(2008): 1504–1509.

Pauker, S. G., and J. P. Kassirer. "Therapeutic Decision Making: A Cost-Benefit Analysis." *N Engl J Med* 293(1975): 229–34.

Paul, D. "Appendix 5: The History of Newborn Phenylketonuria Screening in the U.S." *Promoting Safe and Effective Genetic Testing in the United States,* Final Report of the Task Force on Genetic Testing, September 1997.

Pauly, M. V., and L. R. Burns. "Price Transparency for Medical Devices." *Health Aff (Millwood)* 27(2008): 1544–53.

Pepe, M. S., and T. A. Alonzo. "Comparing Disease Screening Tests When True Disease Status Is Ascertained Only for Screen Positives." *Biostatistics* 2(2001): 249–260.

Petticrew, M., A. Sowden, and D. Lister-Sharp. "False-Negative Results in Screening Programs. Medical, Psychological, and Other Implications." *Int J Technol Assess Health Care* 17(2001): 164–70.

Phillips, K. A. "Closing the Evidence Gap in the Use of Emerging Testing Technologies in Clinical Practice." *JAMA* 300(2008): 2542–44.

Pickhardt, P. J., J. R. Choi, I. Hwang, J. A. Butler, M. L. Puckett, H. A. Hildebrandt, R. K. Wong, P. A. Nugent, P. A. Mysliwiec, and W. R. Schindler. "Computed Tomographic Virtual Colonoscopy to Screen for Colorectal Neoplasia in Asymptomatic Adults." *N Engl J Med* 349(2003): 2191–2200.

Plevritis, S. K. "Decision Analysis and Simulation Modeling for Evaluating Diagnostic Tests on the Basis of Patient Outcomes." *AJR Am J Roentgenol* 185(2005): 581–90.

Pompei, P., M. E. Charlson, and R. G. Douglas. "Clinical Assessments as Predictors of One Year Survival after Hospitalization: Implications for Prognostic Stratification." *J Clin Epidemiol* 41(1988): 275–84.

Pompilio, C. E., and J. E. Vieira. "The Technological Invention of Disease and the Decline of Autopsies." *Sao Paulo Med J* 126(2008): 71–72.

Pray, L. "Gleevec: The Breakthrough in Cancer Treatment." *Nat Educ* 1(2008).

Ransohoff, D. F. "Cancer: Developing Molecular Biomarkers for Cancer." *Science* 299(2003): 1679–80.

Rebbeck, T. R. "Inherited Genetic Markers and Cancer Outcomes: Personalized Medicine in the Postgenome Era." *J Clin Oncol* 24(2006): 1972–74.

Redelmeier, D. A., J. Katz, and D. Kahneman. "Memories of Colonoscopy: A Randomized Trial." *Pain* 104(2003): 187–94.

Reitman, M. L., and E. E. Schadt. "Pharmacogenetics of Metformin Response: A Step in the Path toward Personalized Medicine." *J Clin Invest* 117(2007): 1226–29.

Reyna, V. F. "A Theory of Medical Decision Making and Health: Fuzzy Trace Theory." *Med Decis Making* 28(2008): 850–65.

———. "Theories of Medical Decision Making and Health: An Evidence-Based Approach." *Med Decis Making* 28(2008): 829–33.

"Risky Business." *Nat Genet* 39(2007): 1415.

Roden, D. M., J. M. Pulley, M. A. Basford, G. R. Bernard, E. W. Clayton, J. R. Balser, and D. R. Masys. "Development of a Large-Scale De-Identified DNA Biobank to Enable Personalized Medicine." *Clin Pharmacol Ther* 84(2008): 362–69.

Rose, G., and M. G. Marmot. "Social Class and Coronary Heart Disease." *Br Heart J* 45(1981): 13–19.

Rosenthal, E. T. "Adjuvant! Online Risk-Benefit Profiler: Assessing the Pros and Cons of Letting Patients Have Direct Access." *Oncol Times* 29(2007): 10–15.

Rossouw, J. E., G. L. Anderson, R. L. Prentice, A. Z. LaCroix, C. Kooperberg, M. L. Stefanick, R. D. Jackson, S. A. Beresford, B. V. Howard, K. C. Johnson, J. M. Kotchen, and J. Ockene. "Risks and Benefits of Estrogen Plus Progestin in Healthy Postmenopausal Women: Principal Results from the Women's Health Initiative Randomized Controlled Trial." *JAMA* 288(2002): 321–33.

Rothman, S. *Living in the Shadow of Death: Tuberculosis and the Social Experience of Illness in American History.* Baltimore: Johns Hopkins University Press, 1995.

Rush, A. J. "STAR*D: What Have We Learned?" *Am J Psychiatry* 164(2007): 201–204.

Sankaranarayanan, R., B. M. Nene, S. S. Shastri, K. Jayant, R. Muwonge, A. M. Budukh, S. Hingmire, et al. "HPV Screening for Cervical Cancer in Rural India." *N Engl J Med* 360(2009): 1385–94.

Sattar, N., A. McConnachie, A. G. Shaper, G. J. Blauw, B. M. Buckley, A. J. de Craen, I. Ford, N. G. Forouhi, D. J. Freeman, J. W. Jukema, L. Lennon, P. W. Macfarlane, M. B. Murphy, C. J. Packard, D. J. Stott, R. G. Westendorp, P. H. Whincup, J. Shepherd, and S. G. Wannamethee. "Can Metabolic Syndrome Usefully Predict Cardiovascular Disease and Diabetes? Outcome Data from Two Prospective Studies." *Lancet* 371(2008): 1927–35.

Savitz, D. A. "How Far Can Prenatal Screening Go in Preventing Birth Defects?" *J Pediatr* 152(2008): 3–4.

Scheidt, S., N. Wenger, and M. Weber. "Uncertainty in Medicine: Still Very Much With Us in 2004." *Am J Geriatr Cardiol* 13(2004): 9–10.

Schelling, T. C. "Egonomics, or the Art of Self-Management." *Am Econ Rev* 68(1978): 290–94.

Schlessinger, L., and D. M. Eddy. "Archimedes: A New Model for Simulating Health Care Systems—The Mathematical Formulation." *J Biomed Inform* 35(2002): 37–50.

Schur, C. L., and M. L. Berk. "Views on Health Care Technology: Americans Consider the Risks and Sources of Information." *Health Aff (Millwood)* 27(2008): 1654–64.

Schwartz, A. *Medical Decision Making: A Physician's Guide.* Cambridge, UK: Cambridge University Press, 2008.

Schwartz, L. M., and S. Woloshin. "Participation in Mammography Screening." *BMJ* 335(2007): 731–32.

Schwartz, L. M., S. Woloshin, F. J. Fowler, and H. G. Welch. "Enthusiasm for Cancer Screening in the United States." *JAMA* 291(2004): 71–78.

Schwartz, L. M., S. Woloshin, and H. G. Welch. "Can Patients Interpret Health Information? An Assessment of the Medical Data Interpretation Test." *Med Decis Making* 25(2005): 290–300.

———. "The Drug Facts Box: Providing Consumers with Simple Tabular Data on Drug Benefit and Harm." *Med Decis Making* 27(2007): 655–62.

Schwartz, P. H. "Risk and Disease." *Perspect Biol Med* 51(2008): 320–34.

Scotet, V., B. M. Assael, I. Duguépéroux, A. Tamanini, M. P. Audrezet, C. Férec, and C. Castellani. "Time Trends in Birth Incidence of Cystic Fibrosis in Two European Areas: Data from Newborn Screening Programs." *J Pediatr* 152(2008): 25–32.

Shabo, A. "The Implications of Electronic Health Record for Personalized Medicine." *Biomed Pap Med Fac Univ Palacky Olomouc Czech Repub* 149 Suppl (2005): 251–58.

Shendure, J., G. J. Porreca, N. B. Reppas, X. Lin, J. P. McCutcheon, A. M. Rosenbaum, M. D. Wang, K. Zhang, R. D. Mitra, and G. M. Church. "Accurate Multiplex Polony Sequencing of an Evolved Bacterial Genome." *Science* 309(2005): 1728–32.

Shlipak, M. G., J. H. Ix, K. Bibbins-Domingo, F. Lin, and M. A. Whooley. "Biomarkers to Predict Recurrent Cardiovascular Disease: The Heart and Soul Study." *Am J Med* 121(2008): 50–57.

Shumaker, E. *The Handbook of Health Behavior Change.* 3rd ed. New York: Springer, 2008.

Singman, H. S., S. N. Berman, C. Cowell, E. Maslansky, and M. Archer. "The Anti-Coronary Club: 1957 to 1972." *Am J Clin Nutr* 33(1980): 1183–91.

Skordalakes, E. "Telomerase and the Benefits of Healthy Living." *Lancet Oncol* 9(2008): 1023–1024.

Slack, W. "Computer-Based Interviewing System Dealing with Nonverbal Behavior as Well as Keyboard Responses." *Science* 171(1971): 84–87.

Smedley, B. *Promoting Health Intervention Strategies from Social and Behavioral Research.* Washington, DC: National Academy Press, 2000.

Smith-Bindman, R., D. L. Miglioretti, and E. B. Larson. "Rising Use of Diagnostic Medical Imaging in a Large Integrated Health System." *Health Aff (Millwood)* 27(2008): 1491–1502.

Snyderman, R., and Z. Yoediono. "Perspective: Prospective Health Care and the Role of Academic Medicine: Lead, Follow, or Get Out of the Way." *Acad Med* 83(2008): 707–14.

Spring, B. "Health Decision Making: Lynchpin of Evidence-Based Practice." *Med Decis Making* 28(2008): 866–74.

Stamler, J., and J. Neaton. "The Multiple Risk Factor Intervention Trial (MRFIT)—Importance Then and Now." *JAMA* 300(2008): 1343–45.

Stern, L., N. Iqbal, P. Seshadri, K. L. Chicano, D. A. Daily, J. McGrory, M. Williams, E. J. Gracely, and F. F. Samaha. "The Effects of Low-Carbohydrate versus Conventional Weight Loss Diets in Severely Obese Adults: One-Year Follow-Up of a Randomized Trial." *Ann Intern Med* 140(2004): 778–85.

Stiell, I. G., G. H. Greenberg, R. D. McKnight, R. C. Nair, I. McDowell, and J. R. Worthington. "A Study to Develop Clinical Decision Rules for the Use of Radiography in Acute Ankle Injuries." *Ann Emerg Med* 21(1992): 384–90.

Stiell, I. G., G. H. Greenberg, G. A. Wells, R. D. McKnight, A. A. Cwinn, T. Cacciotti, I. McDowell, and N. A. Smith. "Derivation of a Decision Rule for the Use of Radiography in Acute Knee Injuries." *Ann Emerg Med* 26(1995): 405–13.

Swan, M. "Emerging Patient-Driven Health Care Models: An Examination of Health Social Networks, Consumer Personalized Medicine and Quantified Self-Tracking." *Int J Environ Res Public Health* 6(2009): 492–525.

Tarnawski, A. "Aspirin in the XXI Century: Its Major Clinical Impact, Novel Mechanisms of Action, and New Safer Formulations." *Gastroenterology* 127(2004): 341–43.

Tate, D. F., R. R. Wing, and R. A. Winett. "Using Internet Technology to Deliver a Behavioral Weight Loss Program." *JAMA* 285(2001): 1172–77.

Teunissen, C. E., and P. Scheltens. "Use of Proteomic Approaches to Identify Disease Biomarkers." *Lancet Neurol* 6(2007): 1036–1037.

Thompson, C. "Clinical Experience as Evidence in Evidence-Based Practice." *J Adv Nurs* 43(2003): 230–37.

Thorpe, J. D., X. Duan, R. Forrest, K. Lowe, L. Brown, E. Segal, B. Nelson, G. L. Anderson, M. McIntosh, and N. Urban. "Effects of Blood Collection Conditions on Ovarian Cancer Serum Markers." *PLoS One* 2(2007): e1281.

Toth-Pal, E., I. Wardh, L. E. Strender, and G. Nilsson. "A Guideline-Based Computerised Decision Support System (CDSS) to Influence General

Practitioners Management of Chronic Heart Failure." *Inform Prim Care* 16(2008): 29–39.

Tsai, A. G., and T. A. Wadden. "Systematic Review: An Evaluation of Major Commercial Weight Loss Programs in the United States." *Ann Intern Med* 142(2005): 56–66.

Tsai, S. P., C. P. Wen, H. T. Chan, P. H. Chiang, M. K. Tsai, and T. Y. Cheng. "The Effects of Pre-Disease Risk Factors within Metabolic Syndrome on All-Cause and Cardiovascular Disease Mortality." *Diabetes Res Clin Pract* 82(2008): 148–56.

Tversky, A., and D. Kahneman. "Judgment Under Uncertainty: Heuristics and Biases." *Science* 185(1974): 1124–31.

Varonen, H., T. Kortteisto, and M. Kaila. "What May Help or Hinder the Implementation of Computerized Decision Support Systems (CDSSs): A Focus Group Study with Physicians." *Fam Pract* 25(2008): 162–67.

Vickers, A. J., and E. B. Elkin. "Decision Curve Analysis: A Novel Method for Evaluating Prediction Models." *Med Decis Making* 26(2006): 565–74.

Vickers, A. J., E. B. Elkin, P. B. Peele, M. Dickler, and L. A. Siminoff. "Long-Term Health Outcomes of a Decision Aid: Data from a Randomized Trial of Adjuvant! in Women with Localized Breast Cancer." *Med Decis Making* 29(2009): 461–67.

Vogel, V. G. "Identifying and Screening Patients at Risk of Second Cancers." *Cancer Epidemiol Biomarkers Prev* 15(2006): 2027–2032.

Wakker, P. P. "Lessons Learned by (from?) an Economist Working in Medical Decision Making." *Med Decis Making* 28(2008): 690–98.

Wald, N. J. "All Screening Is Universal." *J Med Screen* 8(2001): 169.

———. "The Definition of Screening." *J Med Screen* 8(2001): 1.

———. "Screening: A Step Too Far. A Matter of Concern." *J Med Screen* 14(2007): 163–64.

Wang, T. J., P. Gona, M. G. Larson, G. H. Tofler, D. Levy, C. Newton-Cheh, P. F. Jacques, N. Rifai, J. Selhub, S. J. Robins, E. J. Benjamin, R. B. D'Agostino, and R. S. Vasan. "Multiple Biomarkers for the Prediction of First Major Cardiovascular Events and Death." *N Engl J Med* 355(2006): 2631–39.

Warner, E., D. B. Plewes, K. A. Hill, P. A. Causer, J. T. Zubovits, R. A. Jong, M. R. Cutrara, G. DeBoer, M. J. Yaffe, S. J. Messner, W. S. Meschino, C. A. Piron, and S. A. Narod. "Surveillance of *BRCA1* and *BRCA2* Mutation Carriers with Magnetic Resonance Imaging, Ultrasound, Mammography, and Clinical Breast Examination." *JAMA* 292(2004): 1317–25.

Weinberg, C. R. "Less Is More, Except When Less Is Less: Studying Joint Effects." *Genomics* 93(2009): 10–12.

Weiss, N. S. "Outcome Events in Studies of Diagnostic or Screening Tests." *J Med Screen* 9(2002): 52–53.

Welch, H. G., L. Schwartz, and S. Woloshin. "What's Making Us Sick Is an

Epidemic of Diagnoses." *New York Times,* January 2, 2007. www.nytimes. com/2007/01/02/health/02essa.html.

Weston, A. D., and L. Hood. "Systems Biology, Proteomics, and the Future of Health Care: Toward Predictive, Preventative, and Personalized Medicine." *J Proteome Res* 3(2004): 179–96.

Weymiller, A. J., V. M. Montori, L. A. Jones, A. Gafni, G. H. Guyatt, S. C. Bryant, T. J. Christianson, R. J. Mullan, and S. A. Smith. "Helping Patients with Type 2 Diabetes Mellitus Make Treatment Decisions: Statin Choice Randomized Trial." *Arch Intern Med* 167(2007): 1076–1082.

Willett, W. "Cancer Prevention and Early Detection." *Cancer Epidemiol Biomarkers Prev* 12(2003): 252s.

Woloshin, S. *Know Your Chances: Understanding Health Statistics.* Berkeley, CA: University of California Press, 2008.

Woloshin, S., L. M. Schwartz, and H. G. Welch. "Patients and Medical Statistics. Interest, Confidence, and Ability." *J Gen Intern Med* 20(2005): 996–1000.

———. "The Effectiveness of a Primer to Help People Understand Risk: Two Randomized Trials in Distinct Populations." *Ann Intern Med* 146(2007): 256–65.

Woolf, S. H. "The Power of Prevention and What It Requires." *JAMA* 299(2008): 2437–39.

Wright, M. O., M. J. Knobloch, C. A. Pecher, G. C. Mejicano, and M. C. Hall. "Clinical Decision Support Systems Use in Wisconsin." *WMJ* 106(2007): 126–29.

Yoon, P. W., M. T. Scheuner, C. Jorgensen, and M. J. Khoury. "Developing Family Healthware, a Family History Screening Tool to Prevent Common Chronic Diseases." *Prev Chronic Dis* 6(2009): A33.

Index

Boldface page references indicate illustrations. <u>Underscored</u> page references indicate charts.